EAT THIS AND LIVE! for KIDS

DON COLBERT, MD
With JOSEPH A. CANNIZZARO, MD

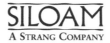

SILOAM
A STRANG COMPANY

Most STRANG COMMUNICATIONS BOOK GROUP products are available at special quantity discounts for bulk purchase for sales promotions, premiums, fund-raising, and educational needs. For details, write Strang Communications Book Group, 600 Rinehart Road, Lake Mary, Florida 32746, or telephone (407) 333-0600.

EAT THIS AND LIVE! FOR KIDS by Don Colbert, MD
Published by Siloam
A Strang Company
600 Rinehart Road
Lake Mary, Florida 32746
www.strangbookgroup.com

Scripture quotations marked NKJV are from the New King James Version of the Bible. Copyright © 1979, 1980, 1982 by Thomas Nelson, Inc., publishers. Used by permission.

Cover design by Nathan Morgan
Design Director: Bill Johnson

Library of Congress Cataloging-in-Publication Data:
An application to register this book for cataloging has been submitted to the Library of Congress.
International Standard Book Number: 978-1-61638-138-7

First Edition

10 11 12 13 14— 9 8 7 6 5 4 3 2 1
Printed in the United States of America

DEDICATION

An article for the prevention of childhood obesity in *Pediatrics*, which is the journal of the American Academy of Pediatrics, states, "Obesity threatens the health of today's children to such an extent that they may, for the first time in U.S. history, have a shorter lifespan than their parents."

Now more than ever, we as parents and grandparents must be an example for our children, grandchildren, and great-grandchildren. Feeding your family is more than just putting food on the table. It's a time to share, nurture, express love, tell stories, and supply healthy foods. It is also a time to teach good eating habits and table manners, to experiment with different foods, and to praise your children for making healthy choices.

Deuteronomy 4 tells us to teach our children and grandchildren. Verse 5 says, "Behold, I have taught you statutes and judgments, even as the Lord my God commanded me." Verse 9 tells us to teach them to our sons and sons' sons. We must lead by example, because whether we realize it or not, our children will model our eating behavior and food choices.

I dedicate this book to my grandchildren: Caleb, Jarret, Kate, Olen, and Braden, and to my future grandchildren (one is on the way right now). In teaching them to make the correct food choices, my hope is that they will in turn teach their children and grandchildren the same.

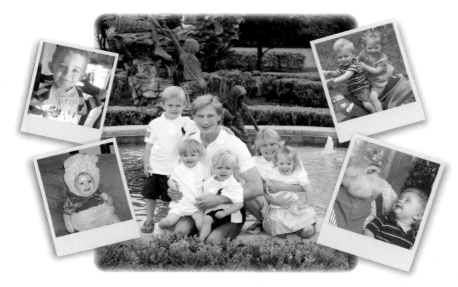

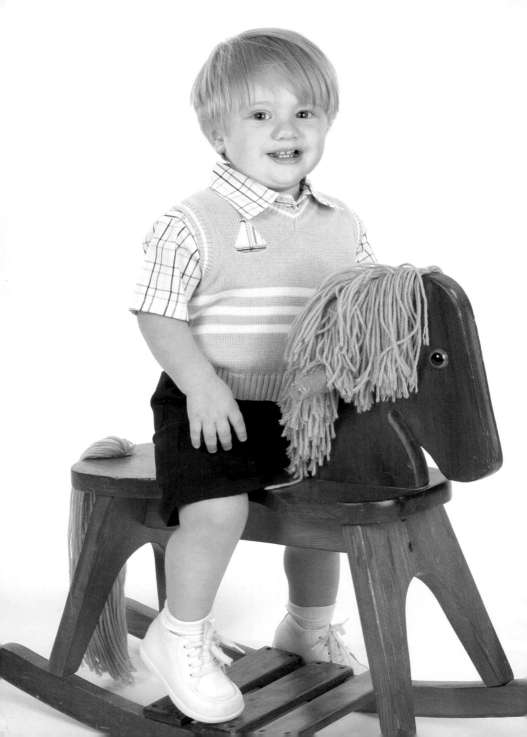

CONTENTS

INTRODUCTION

from Don Colbert, MD

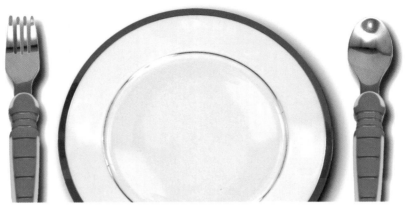

For the first time in two hundred years, children in America may have a shorter life expectancy than their parents. The reason? Obesity! A report in the *New England Journal of Medicine* predicts that the rise in childhood obesity could reduce the lifespan of this current generation of children by five years.[1] All parents know what a challenge it can be to get kids to enjoy healthy foods at times. But in light of the epidemic of childhood obesity we're facing, teaching kids to eat living foods is one of the most important things parents can do.

When I wrote *The Seven Pillars of Health*, I introduced people to the seven basic pillars of a healthy lifestyle. I believe that by living out the seven principles I shared in that book, anyone can become stronger, healthier, more energetic, younger-looking, wiser, smarter, and more disease-resistant. The third pillar of *The Seven Pillars of Health* lays the groundwork to help you obtain a deeper understanding of why some foods are healthy ("living") and some are unhealthy ("dead"). Using this groundwork, we created *Eat This and Live!* and now *Eat This and Live! for Kids*.

As a medical doctor who is board certified in family practice and anti-aging medicine, I have dedicated my life to helping people become healthy. Because I have spent more than twenty years treating patients, the advice I give in my books is based on my years of experience with real problems and real people.

One area of health that I commonly address when treating my patients is their diet. But as I mentioned, with childhood obesity and obesity-related illnesses on the rise, it is becoming more and more critical that parents also address the dietary choices of their children. The key is knowing what foods to feed your children heartily, what foods to give in moderation, and what foods to avoid. Wouldn't it be great if there were a road map to help you as a parent to navigate through the often-treacherous territory of healthy food choices? That is exactly what you hold in your hands.

Eat This and Live! for Kids is written for parents who want to help their children establish healthy eating patterns to last a lifetime. To make sure I've provided you with the latest and most cutting-edge advice for children's health, I've asked a colleague of mine, Joseph A. Cannizzaro, MD, to contribute to this book based on his decades of experience as a pediatrician who, like me, approaches treatment from an integrative, whole-person perspective.

I've also provided you with my picks of the healthiest "kid-friendly" food items in your grocery store and many popular fast food and casual dining restaurants. As a result, this is an extremely practical guidebook that teaches you how to help your child adopt a dietary lifestyle that will set him or her on a lifelong path of well-being. My goal is not to make eating a chore for you or your child, or to make more work on your part, but to enable you to exchange old habits for new ones.

Meet Joseph A. Cannizzaro, MD

For the past twenty years, Dr. Joseph Cannizzaro and I have been referring patients to each other. As a pediatrician whose practice is located just a few miles from mine in Longwood, Florida, he and I are very like-minded in our approach to medicine—combining the best of both traditional and alternative treatments that address a person's body, mind, and spirit. That's why Dr. Cannizzaro was my first and only choice as a contributing author when I embarked upon creating a book that focuses on healthy eating and lifestyle choices for children. I encourage you to read Appendix A, where he shares his background and perspective on nutritional health.

EATING HABITS OF THE NEXT GENERATION

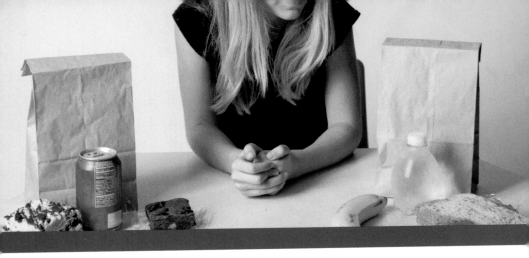

EATING HABITS
AND OUR FUTURE

HOW HAS AN ENTIRE generation of hefty eaters changed the face of the world? By starting young. And once again, this unflattering trend originated in America. In the United States, 17.1 percent of our children and adolescents—that's 2.5 million youth—are now reported to be obese.[1] Obesity in children has risen from less than 5 percent in 1980 to 17 percent in 2006.[2] According to the Institute of Medicine, between 1960 and 2000, childhood obesity has more than tripled in children between the ages of six and eleven, and more than doubled for children between the ages of two and five.[3]

As a result of childhood obesity, we are seeing a dramatic rise in type 2 diabetes throughout the country. And because of the connection obesity has with hypertension, hypercholesterolemia (high cholesterol), and heart disease, experts are predicting a dramatic rise in heart disease as our children become adults. The Centers for Disease Control and Prevention (CDC) reports that overweight teens stand a 70 percent chance of becoming overweight adults, and that is increased to 80 percent if at least one parent is overweight or obese. Because of that, heart disease, type 2 diabetes, fatty liver, high blood pressure, high cholesterol, acid reflux disease, and obstructive sleep apnea are expected to begin at a much earlier age in those who fail to beat the odds.[4] Overall, this is the first generation of children that is not expected to live as long as their parents, and they will be more likely to suffer from disease and illness.

If you do not take charge of your food choices for yourself, at least do it for your children. Children follow by example, by mirroring the behavior of their parents. Don't tell them to make healthy eating choices without doing it yourself. I'm sure most of you love your children and are good parents. But ask yourself: Do you love your children enough to make the necessary lifestyle changes? Do you love them enough to educate them on what foods to eat and what foods to avoid? Do you love them enough to keep junk food out of your house and instead make healthy food more available? Do you love them enough to exercise regularly and lead by example?

If you answered yes to those questions, it is important that you not only take action right now but also that you make changes for them that last a lifetime.

But let me be honest; this is not an easy fight when it involves your children's lives. As the little boxes of information on this page illustrate, the culture in which your children are growing up is saturated with junk food that is void of nutrition but high in inflammatory fats, sugars, highly processed carbohydrates, and food additives. Consuming these foods has become part of childhood.

You can do it, but you must be prepared to stand strong! That's why I am ecstatic that you have picked up this book. I believe you now hold a key to truly changing your life and your children's lives.

Stand Strong!

If you're planning on taking a stand against this garbage-in, garbage-out culture, expect some opposition from every front. During the course of a year, the typical American child will watch more than thirty thousand television commercials, with many of these advertisements pitching fast-food or junk food as delicious "must-eats." For years, fast food franchises have enticed children into their restaurants with kids' meal toys, promotional giveaways, and elaborate playgrounds. It has obviously worked for McDonald's: about 90 percent of American children between the ages of three and nine set foot in one each month.[5]

It's All Part of the Plan

Fast-food establishments spend billions of dollars on research and marketing. They know exactly what they are doing and how to push your child's hot button. They understand the powerful impact certain foods can have. That is why comfort foods often do more than just fill the stomach; they bring about memories of the fair, playgrounds, toys, backyard birthday bashes, Fourth of July parties, childhood friends…the list goes on. Advertisers have keyed into this and learned to use the sight of food to stimulate the same fond childhood memories.

School Cafeteria or Fast Food Franchise?

When your kids can't visit the Golden Arches, it comes to them. Fast-food products—most of which are brought in by franchises—are sold in about 30 percent of public high school cafeterias and many elementary cafeterias.[6] According to researchers at the U.S. Department of Agriculture (USDA), on a typical day, 30 percent of children consume fast food.[7]

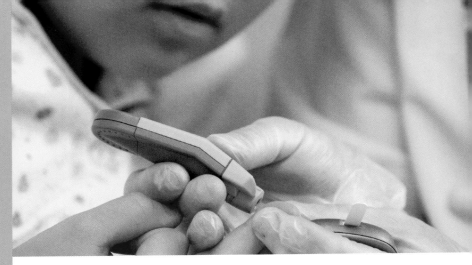

AN ALARMING TREND IN CHILDREN'S HEALTH

BY TEACHING YOUR CHILDREN healthy eating habits, you can keep them at a healthy weight. Also, the eating habits your children pick up when they are young will help them maintain a healthy lifestyle when they are adults. The challenges we face are imposing. The state of children's health today is, according to recent measures, at its most dire. The rise in rates of complex, chronic childhood disorders has been well profiled. Here are some concrete examples of the current state of children's health:

- Cancer remains the leading cause of death by disease in children, with the most common cases being leukemia and cancers of the brain and nervous system.[8]

- Obesity is epidemic. Research shows that from 1980 to 2006 the prevalence of obesity has jumped from 5 percent to 12 percent in children ages two to five, from 6.5 percent to 17 percent in ages six to eleven, and from 5 percent to 17.6 percent in ages twelve to nineteen.[9]

- Twenty percent of children are overweight.[10]

- Diabetes now affects 1 in every 500 children. Of those children newly diagnosed with diabetes, the percentage with type 2 ("adult-onset") has risen from less than 5 percent to nearly 50 percent in a ten-year period.[11]

- Asthma is the most prevalent chronic disease affecting American children, leading to 15 million missed days of school per year. Since 1980, the percentage of children with asthma has almost tripled.[12]

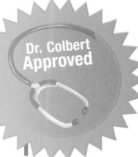

Dr. Colbert
Approved

EAT THIS AND LIVE! For Kids

Top Three Tips for Parents

1. Lead by example. Your child will have an extremely difficult time making healthy eating choices and exercising regularly if you don't consistently show him or her how. Numerous studies have shown that parents' dietary and exercise choices and behavior have a powerful influence on a child's weight as he or she grows and develops.

2. Take baby steps that lead to lasting changes. If your child is overweight, avoid diets that promise instant weight loss. Gradual changes that move your family toward more healthful living are a better way to go.

3. Take your time as you replace your child's old habits with healthy ones. This goes hand in hand with tip #2. You're in this for the long haul. It takes time to adapt to a new lifestyle. Be patient as he or she adjusts to the new eating habits and activities that you will be introducing.

- Approximately 1 in 25 American children now suffer from food allergies. From 1997 to 2007, the prevalence of reported food allergy increased 18 percent among children under the age of eighteen years.[13]

- One in 6 children is diagnosed with a significant neurodevelopmental disability, including 1 in 12 with ADHD. Autism affects 1 in 110 U.S. children, an extraordinary rise in prevalence.[14]

- Babies in one study were noted, at birth, to have an average of 200 industrial chemicals and pollutants present in their umbilical cord blood.[15]

These statistics are sobering indeed, and perhaps the most sobering is the rise in childhood obesity. Why? Obesity plays a part in several other chronic illnesses that are also on the rise among children. And there's an unwelcome side effect—more kids are being put on prescription medications for obesity-related chronic diseases. Across the board, we are witnessing increases in prescriptions for children with high blood pressure, high cholesterol, type 2 diabetes, depression, attention-deficit/hyperactivity disorder, and asthma. There must be a better way.

What we need now is an absolute paradigm shift. No longer are the "one drug, one disease" solutions of the past appropriate. These are times that demand out-of-the-box thinking. That's where this book can help. If your child is overweight or you want to lower his or her risk of becoming overweight down the road, there are many positive, natural ways you can address the situation. In this book, Dr. Cannizzaro and I provide you with information and ideas to help you help your child.

Understanding Childhood Obesity

NOW THAT WE'VE SHARED the bad news about the childhood obesity epidemic in the United States, let's make sure you really understand the terms *overweight* and *obese*. Many people have a general sense as to how these words are different, yet in recent years the delineation has become clearer. Various health organizations, including the CDC and the National Institutes of Health (NIH), now officially define these terms using the body mass index (BMI), which factors in a person's weight relative to height. Most of these organizations define an overweight adult (twenty years of age and older) as having a BMI between 25 and 29.9, while an obese adult is anyone who has a BMI of 30 or higher.[16]

For children and teens, BMI is measured differently, allowing for the normal variations in body composition between boys and girls and at various ages. For ages two to nineteen, the BMI (or BMI-for-age) is pinpointed on a growth chart to determine the corresponding age- and sex-specific percentile.

- Overweight is defined as a BMI at or above the 85th percentile and lower than the 95th percentile.

- Obesity is defined as a BMI at or above the 95th percentile for children of the same age and sex.

BMI is the most widely accepted method used to determine body fat in children and adults because it's easy to measure a person's height and weight. However, while BMI is an acceptable screening tool for initial assessment of body composition, please remember that it is not a direct measure of body fatness. There are other factors that can affect body composition, and your child's doctor can discuss these with you.

If you think your child may be overweight, start by talking to his or her pediatrician. (See the box on the next page for some suggested questions to ask your child's doctor.) After determining your child's BMI and targeting a healthy weight range for your child, make a plan together as a family. It's a good idea to include any regular caregivers in this plan as well. Set a goal for the whole family to get lots of activity and eat a healthy, well-balanced diet.

Wondering About Your Child's Weight?
Five Questions to Ask Your Pediatrician

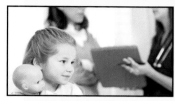

I understand that you probably don't want to talk about the possibility that your child may not be at a healthy weight. To help make this as painless as possible, I recommend asking your doctor the following questions to get the conversation started.

1. *What is a healthy weight for my child's height?* Your doctor will use a growth chart to show you how your child is growing and give you a healthy weight range for your child. The doctor may also tell you your child's body mass index (BMI).

2. *Is my child's weight putting him or her at risk for any illnesses?* Based on your family history and other factors, your doctor can help you to determine what health risks your child may be facing. Overweight and obese inactive children have an increased risk of being diagnosed with type 2 diabetes. High blood pressure and all the diseases listed on pages 7–8 can also occur in overweight children.

3. *How much exercise does my child need?* The National Association for Sport and Physical Education, the 2005 Dietary Guidelines for Americans, and the U.S. Department of Health and Human Services all recommend at least one hour of moderate or vigorous intensity physical activity or exercise a day. However, according to the CDC, only 35 percent of children engage in any kind of physical activity that raises their heart and breathing rates.[17] Talk to your doctor and see chapter 9 for specific ways to help increase your child's activity level.

4. *Does my child need to go on a diet?* Although an overweight and obese child's eating habits will need to change, I don't advise using the word *diet* because it focuses on short-term eating habits that are rarely sustainable for long-term health. Children (and adults) who become chronic dieters are setting themselves up for problems with their metabolism later in life. Researchers at the University of Minnesota found that teens who were pressured to diet are three times more likely to be carrying excess weight five years later.[18] A healthier approach—including a healthy breakfast, healthy beverages, and quality time at dinner—is to put your whole family on the path to healthy food choices and portion sizes with gradual but permanent changes.

5. *How do I talk about weight without hurting my child's feelings?* Above all, the message must never be, "You're fat," or "You need to lose weight." Instead, it should be praising your child for healthy food choices and providing unconditional love with plenty of hugs, kisses, and quality time. Tell your child that you'll always love his or her body and that you will love him or her at any size. Say, "Our family needs to make better choices about eating and being more active so that we all can be healthy."

DON COLBERT, MD | 10

WHY FOOD CHOICES MATTER

All men are created equal, but all foods are not! In fact, some food should not be labeled "food" but rather "consumable product" or "edible, but void of nourishment."

Living foods—fruits, vegetables, grains, seeds, and nuts—exist in a raw or close-to-raw state and are beautifully packaged in divinely created wrappers called skins and peels. Living foods look robust, healthy, and alive. They have not been bleached, refined, or chemically enhanced and preserved. Living foods are plucked, harvested, and squeezed—not processed, packaged, and put on a shelf.

Dead foods are the opposite. They have been altered in every imaginable way to make them last as long as possible and be as addictive as possible. That usually means the manufacturer adds considerable amounts of sugar, salt, and man-made fats that involve taking various oils and heating them to high temperatures so that the nutrients die and the oils are inflammatory and toxic to our bodies.

Life breeds life. Death breeds death. When your child eats living foods, the enzymes in their pristine state interact with his or her digestive enzymes. The other natural ingredients God put in them—vitamins, minerals, phytonutrients, antioxidants, fiber, and more—flow into your child's system in their natural state. These living foods were created to cause your child's digestive system, immune system, and organs and tissues to function at optimum capacity.

Dead foods hit your child's body like a foreign intruder. Chemicals, including preservatives, food additives, and bleaching agents, may place a strain on the liver. Toxic man-made fats begin to form in your child's cell membranes; they become stored as fat in your child's body and start the process of forming plaque in his or her arteries. Your child's body does its best to harvest the tiny traces of good from these nutrient-depleted or dead foods, but in the end he or she usually is undernourished and overweight.

If you want your child to be a healthy, energetic person rather than someone struggling with their weight for the rest of their life, begin to take his or her eating habits seriously. Now is the time to help your son or daughter make the change to more living foods.

Isn't It Really Just Genetics?

For every obese person, there is a story behind the excessive weight gain. Growing up, I would often hear it said of an obese person that "she was just born fat," or "he takes after his daddy." There's some truth in both of those. Genetics count when it comes to obesity.

In 1988, the *New England Journal of Medicine* published a Danish study that observed five hundred forty people who had been adopted during infancy. The research found that adopted individuals had a much greater tendency to end up in the weight class of their biological parents rather than their adopted parents.[19] Separate studies have proven that twins who were raised apart also reveal that genes have a strong influence on gaining weight or becoming overweight.[20] There is a significant genetic predisposition to gaining weight.

Still, that does not fully explain the epidemic of obesity seen in the United States over the past thirty years. Although an individual may have a genetic predisposition to become obese, environment plays a major role as well. I like the way author, speaker, and noted women's physician Pamela Peeke said

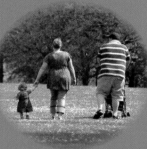

it: "Genetics may load the gun, but environment pulls the trigger."[21] Many patients I see come into my office thinking they have inherited their "fat genes," and therefore there is nothing they can do about it. After investigating a little, I usually find that they simply inherited their parents' propensity for bad choices of foods, large portion sizes, and poor eating habits.

Also realize that our genetic makeup hasn't changed significantly over the generations, but our environmental influences have changed dramatically. Fast food, junk food, sodas, large portion sizes, lack of activity, and commercials touting the above have accelerated the obesity epidemic.

If your child is overweight, he or she may have an increased number of fat cells, which means your child will have a tendency to gain weight if you choose to provide the wrong types of foods, large portion sizes, and allow him or her to be inactive. But you should also realize that most people can override their genetic makeup for obesity by making the correct dietary and lifestyle choices. Unfortunately, many parents forget that to make these healthy choices, it helps to surround a child with a healthy environment and to be a model of the lifestyle as well.

2

THE BASICS OF GOOD NUTRITION

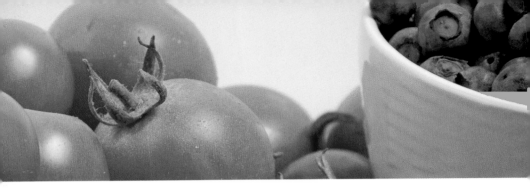

THE POWER OF ANTIOXIDANTS FROM FRUITS AND VEGETABLES

BEFORE DISCUSSING ANTIOXIDANTS, YOU must understand free radicals. Free radicals are formed by a chemical process called oxidation. If you were to leave a brand-new iron pipe outside in the elements, within a short period of time rust would occur. Rust is due to oxidation and free radicals. When oxidation occurs on painted surfaces, the paint begins to flake. When you cut an apple in half, it begins to turn brown within minutes due to oxidation.

Free radicals are produced in our bodies simply by breathing. When our cells produce energy in the form of ATP, free radicals referred to as reactive oxygen species are also produced.

Free radicals are very damaging to cell membranes; cellular components, including the mitochondria (where energy is produced); and nuclear membranes. Everyone forms free radicals; the problem arises when too many free radicals are produced and/or when an individual has inadequate antioxidant protection to neutralize the free radicals.

Excessive free radicals are produced by eating too many inflammatory foods, which I will be discussing. Excessive amounts are also produced from smoking, toxic exposure, drugs, chemicals, emotional stress, excessive exercise, sunlight, radiation, and so on. The problem arises when excessive amounts of free radicals overwhelm the body's antioxidants, and chronic inflammation usually results. Allergies, asthma, and chronic infections are all inflammatory conditions.

The body has a natural defense against free radicals: antioxidants. One of the antioxidants your child's body produces is glutathione, which neutralizes free radicals.

Your primary antioxidant source is your foods—especially fruits and vegetables. It is clearly best for your health to quench free radicals with antioxidants to prevent excessive free-radical damage from pushing the body into an inflammatory state that can eventually lead to disease.

Among the many antioxidants supplied by fruits and vegetables are:

- Vitamin E and the carotenoid beta-carotene defend cell membranes from free-radical damage.

- Vitamin C protects the body's watery components; it neutralizes free radicals from polluted air and cigarette smoke.

- Green leafy vegetables such as spinach and kale contain lutein, another powerful carotenoid antioxidant that protects the eyes against cataracts and macular degeneration.

- Many minerals are antioxidants as well.

- Iodine helps prevent lipid peroxidation.

- The mineral selenium is a component of the antioxidant glutathione peroxidase, which protects red blood cells and cell membranes from free radicals by working in conjunction with vitamin E.

The antioxidant and phytonutrient properties you get in fruits and vegetables cannot be found anywhere else. Experts recommend that everyone, both children and adults, eat at least five servings of fruits and vegetables a day. The portion size should be based on the person's age.

According to Dr. William Castelli, director of the Framingham Heart Study, "A low-fat plant-based diet would not only lower the heart attack rate about 85 percent, but would lower the cancer rate 60 percent."[1]

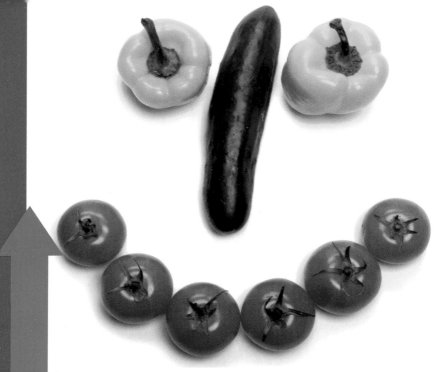

PHYTONUTRIENTS AND PARTICULARLY POWERFUL FOODS

IT SEEMS TOO SIMPLE to be true, but when you realize that each fruit and vege-table contains hundreds of thousands of known and unknown phytochemicals, you can better understand the power of whole foods. It is always best to eat the whole food to get all of its synergistic phytochemicals and nutrients in nature's normal optimal balance.

Whole foods supply a cornucopia of beneficial compounds in a synergistic balance that can never be duplicated by man. Raw foods that are not processed or cooked have a God-given balance that coexists as interconnected food elements: vitamins, minerals, antioxidants, phytonutrients, enzymes, proteins, carbohydrates, and fats.

Phytonutrients At-a-Glance

Phenols reduce oxidative stress.

Flavonoids are anti-inflammatory and protect against allergic reactions.

Quercetin protects against heart disease and allergies and reduces inflammation in sports injuries.

Phytosteroids block the development of breast, colon, and prostate diseases.

Carotenoids stimulate the immune system.

Lycopene helps prevent prostate cancer.

Lutein protects against macular degeneration, the leading cause of blindness and cataracts.

Zeaxanthin protects against developing blindness.

Ellagic acid is a cancer fighter.

Indoles are more fighters against cancer.

Sulforaphane prevents colon cancer.

Anthocyanidins strengthen the collagen protein in soft tissues, tendons, ligaments, and bones.

Catechins are antioxidant flavonoids found in green tea.

Citrus fruits contain phytochemicals with antitumor and antioxidant properties.

Flaxseed, a good source of omega-3 fats, lowers cholesterol and can inhibit the growth of estrogen-stimulated breast cancers.

Red wine and grape juice contain phenols and red anthocyanins that protect against heart disease.

Garlic and onions are rich in allylsulfides, which reduce cancer risk and blood clotting.

What Are Phytonutrients or Phytochemicals?

Phyto- means "plant," so phyto-chemicals or phytonutrients are found naturally in fruits, vegetables, seeds, nuts, and legumes. They naturally protect their plants against viruses, bacteria, and fungi. As a result, they act as scavengers of free radicals in our cells, slow the aging process, strengthen the immune system, and reduce the risk of cancer and heart disease.

Cooking and processing foods can destroy phyto-chemicals. Some do remain in cooked foods, but the best way to get them in their most useful form is to eat raw or slightly steamed vegetables and fruits.

The optimal function of any of these chemicals depends on the presence of the chemicals normally found along with it. That's why vitamins and minerals taken by themselves some-times just don't seem to work. When individual nutrients are taken, they will not act the same as when you eat them in whole food. Therefore, your child needs both supplements and whole foods.

THE ANTI-INFLAMMATORY DIET

THE MAJORITY OF CHILDHOOD diseases are inflammatory diseases. All infections—such as otitis media, pharyngitis, tonsillitis, bronchitis, sinusitis, and other infections—are inflammatory. Also, obesity, and especially belly fat, is typically inflammatory and is associated with elevated CRP levels, a marker of inflammation. Other common inflammatory diseases in children include eczema, dermatitis, asthma, and allergies. Chronic inflammation is also associated with autoimmune diseases, cancer, and heart disease.

In fact, inflammation is at the root of most pediatric diseases. Inflammation refers to the redness, swelling, pain, and warmth that occur when an area of the body is inflamed. An injury, such as a sprained ankle, is simply inflammation in the ankle, and the ankle is usually red, swollen, painful, and warm. A foreign body, such as a splinter in your finger, causes inflammation. An infection, such as tonsillitis from the strep bacterium, causes inflammation. This is the good side of inflammation, which enables the body to fight infection or splint an injury or wall off a foreign body such as a splinter, preventing it from infecting the entire body.

The bad side of inflammation occurs when inflammation is not turned off and continues long term, such as in allergies, asthma, eczema, chronic ear infections, chronic sinusitis, chronic mono, and other chronic infections. Eating inflammatory foods such as sugars, high-glycemic foods, toxic and inflammatory oils and fats, fried foods, and foods that you may be allergic or sensitive to will typically fan the flames of inflammation. For example, many children with chronic ear infections are sensitive to dairy and improve significantly when dairy is eliminated. Also, inhalant allergies to dust, mold, pollen, and animal dander can increase inflammation in the body.

Chronic degenerative diseases (CDD) result from extended periods (years) of low-level inflammation. CDD includes all cancers, heart disease, diabetes, neurodegenerative diseases (Alzheimer's), and obesity. Acute or short-term inflammation is the cornerstone of the body's healing response (it's powerful), but chronic or long-term inflammation is very damaging to the body, and usually, it eventually leads to disease.

Your child's body regulates inflammation through a very complex, coordinated pattern of opposing biochemical forces. A balance is needed between hormone regulating compounds that either up-regulate or down-regulate inflammation. If you can't mount a good inflammatory response, you're at risk for infections. If it's excessive and you can't turn it off, you're at risk for tissue damage, which can lead to allergies or autoimmunity. Cancer is related to up-regulation of inflammation, where overstimulation of cells occurs, increasing the risk of malignant transformation. Chronic degenerative diseases usually all have one common root: excess inflammation. This should help you understand why it is so important to regulate inflammation. And the good news is that feeding your child an anti-inflammatory diet goes a long way in keeping inflammation at bay.

Carbohydrates

Carbohydrates are critical for good health, but most carbs have received a bad rap over the years.

The important thing to remember is how carbohydrates are digested and how they impact your child's blood sugar levels. Scientists can measure how rapidly carbs are converted into glucose in the bloodstream; this measurement is called the glycemic index. A food with a high-glycemic score has a very rapid rate of converting into glucose.

The main driver of obesity in children is the way we have transformed carbohydrate foods. We've taken whole grains and made them into white bread, a high-glycemic food, causing dramatic shifts in blood glucose levels in genetically susceptible people. Rapidly digested foods and beverages are more prone to be stored as fat due to elevated insulin levels that program the body to store fat.

Whole grains are healthier for your child. Why? Because they are digested slowly (low glycemic), have a higher fiber content, and generally do not raise the blood sugar significantly.

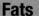

Protein

Protein is needed for cellular structure, repair, maintenance, and growth. Children are growing and require adequate amounts of protein with each meal to build strong tissues, organs, and a strong immune system. Choose organic or free-range chicken breast without the skin, turkey breast, lean red meats, Alaskan salmon, and tongol tuna instead of processed meats such as bologna, bacon, sausage, pepperoni, spam, salami, and others. Do not deep-fry. As a guideline, serve 1 tablespoon of protein for each year of age for children five years old or younger.

Fats

We need to consume approximately 30 percent of our total calories from fat if our diet is high in antioxidant foods and if we use more monounsaturated fats from olives and nuts and consume adequate essential fatty acids (omega 3s and modest amounts of omega 6s).

We can safely consume about 10 percent of our calories as saturated fats if these preconditions are met. Low-fat cheese made from the organic milk of free-range cows usually has a good essential fatty acids profile. You can ensure your child is not exceeding the 10 percent range for saturated fats by choosing extra-lean cuts of meat, peeling the skins off of poultry, and limiting red meat to two or three times a week.

Most Americans consume an anti-inflammatory diet with excessive omega-6 (inflammatory) fats and insufficient omega-3 (anti-inflammatory) fats. Ideal ratios of omega 6 to omega 3 should be 4:1, but the standard American diet is about 30:1. To bring this ratio into balance, foods rich in omega 3 must be eaten (such as flaxseeds, wild salmon, and pharmaceutical-grade fish oil).

INFLAMMATORY AND ANTI-INFLAMMATORY FOODS

I HIGHLY RECOMMEND MONICA Reinagel's *The Inflammation Free Diet Plan,* where she presents her years of research to ascribe an Inflammation Free (IF) Rating to the foods we eat. This rating system takes into account more than twenty different factors that contribute to a food's relationship to inflammation. Positive ratings are anti-inflammatory, and foods with negative ratings promote inflammation. Up to a hundred on each scale is considered mildly one way or the other, over a hundred is moderate, and over five hundred is severe.

Looking at her research and adding some of my own, I have organized the following two lists of foods for you to consider adding or subtracting from your child's diet as his or her level of inflammation demands.

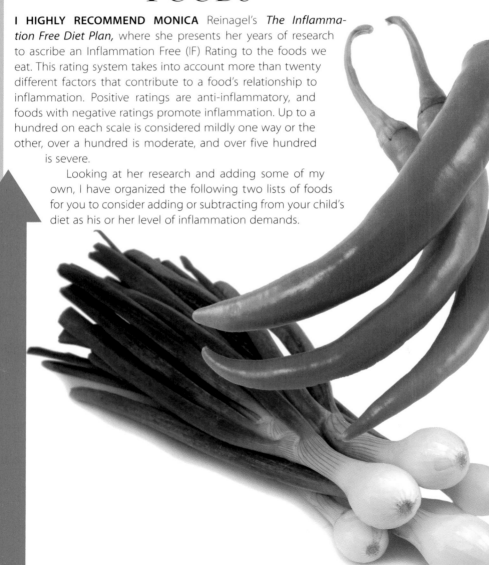

Top Anti-Inflammatory Foods (Always Choose Organic When Possible)

Fruit	Raspberries, acerola (West Indian) cherries, guava, strawberries, cantaloupe, lemons/limes, rhubarb, kumquat, pink grapefruit, mulberries
Vegetables	Chili peppers, onions (including scallions and leeks), spinach, greens (including kale, collards, turnip, and mustard greens), sweet potatoes, carrots, garlic
Legumes	Lentils, green beans
Egg Products	Liquid eggs, egg whites
Dairy	Cottage cheese (low fat and nonfat), nonfat cream cheese, margarine (soy or cottonseed), plain yogurt
Fish	Herring, mackerel (not king), wild salmon (not farmed; Alaskan preferred), rainbow trout, sardines, anchovies
Poultry (Remove Skin)	Goose, duck, free-range organic chicken and turkey (white meat)
Lean Meat (limit to 18 ounces or less per week)	Pot roast, beef shank, eye of round (beef), flank steak, sirloin tip, prime rib, skirt steak, pork rib chops, pork tenderloin
Cereal	All-Bran, Total, bran flakes
Breads/Pasta	Ezekiel 4:9 bread, sprouted breads, whole-wheat spaghetti (thick noodles), brown rice pasta, couscous, buckwheat groats, barley
Fats/Oils	Safflower oil (high oleic), hazelnut oil, olive oil, avocado oil, almond oil, apricot kernel oil, cod liver oil, macadamia nut oil, flaxseed oil (do not cook with this)
Nuts/Seeds	Brazil nuts, macadamia nuts, hazelnuts, pecans, almonds, hickory nuts, cashews, flaxseeds
Herbs/Spices	Garlic, onion, cayenne, ginger, turmeric, chili peppers, chili powder, curry powder
Sweeteners	Stevia
Beverages	Carrot juice, tomato juice, black or green tea, club soda/seltzer, herbal tea, spring water

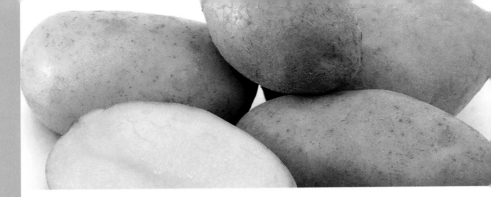

INFLAMMATORY AND ANTI-INFLAMMATORY FOODS (CONT'D)

	Inflammatory Foods to Limit or Avoid
Fruit	Mango, banana, dried apricots, dried apples, dried dates, canned fruits, raisins (this refers to excessive amounts of these fruits)
Vegetables	Corn, white potatoes, french fries
Legumes	Baked beans, fava beans (boiled), canned beans
Egg Products	Duck eggs, goose eggs, hard-boiled eggs, egg yolks
Cheeses	Most all high-fat cheeses, including brick cheese, cheddar cheese, Colby cheese, cream cheese (normal and reduced fat)
Dairy	Flavored or fruit-on-the-bottom yogurt, ice cream, butter, whole milk, 2 percent milk, whipping cream
Fish	Farmed salmon and other farm-raised fish, swordfish, tilefish, tuna, halibut, sea bass, bluefish, king mackerel
Poultry	Turkey (dark meat), Cornish game hen, chicken giblets, chicken liver, chicken (dark meat)
Meat	All processed meats and organ meats, bacon, all veal (loin and shank), pork chitterlings, all lamb (rib, chops, shanks, loin), pork ribs and shoulder roast
Breads	Hot dog/hamburger buns, english muffins, kaiser rolls, bagels, french bread, vienna bread, blueberry muffins, oat bran muffins
Cereal	Grape-Nuts, Crispix, Corn Chex, Just Right, Rice Chex, corn flakes, Rice Krispies, Raisin Bran, shredded wheat
Pasta/Grain	White rice, millet, corn pasta, cornmeal, lasagna noodles, macaroni elbows, angel hair and regular spaghetti pasta

Inflammatory Foods to Limit or Avoid	
Fats/Oils	Margarine, wheat germ oil, sunflower oil, poppy seed oil, grape seed oil, safflower oil, cottonseed oil, palm kernel oil, coconut oil, corn oil
Nuts/Seeds	Poppy seeds, walnuts, pine nuts, sunflower seeds
Sweeteners	Honey, brown sugar, white sugar, corn syrup, powdered sugar, agave nectar
Crackers/Chips/Cookies	All cookies, chips, and crackers, including corn chips, pretzels, graham crackers, saltines, vanilla wafers, potato chips
Desserts	Sweetened condensed milk, angel food cake, chocolate and vanilla cake with frosting, chocolate chips, whipped cream, ice cream, fruit leather snacks
Candy	All candy, including chocolate Kisses, jelly beans, Twix, Almond Joy, milk chocolate bars, Snickers
Beverages	All fruit juices and sodas, Gatorade, lemonade, sugar-laden soft drinks, commercial smoothies, and coffee drinks

These are not complete lists by any means—just some of the more likely "suspects" to watch out for or some of the more helpful helpers to work into your child's diet. As you read these now, some of these will jump out at you as things your child likes and needs, but needs more of in his or her diet. Or maybe they are the foods that you know it is time to change your child's habits about and say good-bye to. The thing to remember is that you make the majority of the choices about what your child puts in his or her mouth, and now that you have a little more knowledge about these foods, you can begin making healthier diet choices concerning them.

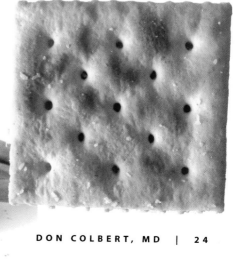

A HEALTHY BABY
DURING PREGNANCY

A HEALTHY BABY BEGINS WITH A HEALTHY DIET

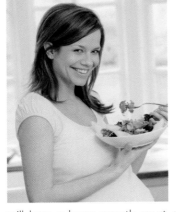

IDEALLY, A WOMAN SHOULD begin paying attention to certain nutrients, like folic acid, before she becomes pregnant. A healthy diet including a variety of foods not only enhances fertility but also provides the nourishment a developing embryo needs during the critical early days after conception.

During the first few weeks of pregnancy, your baby needs an adequate supply of essential nutrients, since this is when all the cells form that will develop into your baby's organs. After the first trimester, some of your baby's specific nutritional needs change. For example, calcium is especially important during the second trimester, when bone and blood development escalates. In the last trimester, your baby will have a huge growth spurt, nearly doubling in size, so more protein is required.

Studies in humans and animals indicate that nutrition during pregnancy influences not only the normal development of the fetus and immediate health of the newborn infant, but there are now also compelling data that nutrition during pregnancy influences your child's health and longevity as a grown adult.[1]

Current recommendations for nutrition during pregnancy stress the importance of a proper pattern of weight gain and an adequate intake of calories, protein, vitamins, and minerals to allow for optimal development of your baby and the preservation of your own health. Physicians typically recommend an average weight gain of 25 to 35 pounds during pregnancy—more if you are underweight to begin with. For patients who are overweight, an average of 15 to 25 pounds is recommended, and for patients who are underweight, the recommended average weight gain is 28 to 40 pounds.

A woman's estimated energy requirements gradually increase during her pregnancy to an additional 450 calories per day in the third trimester. If you are pregnant, it is recommended that you consume an additional 20 grams of protein a day to support the deposition of protein in the new maternal and fetal tissues.

If you are a vegetarian—particularly if you do not eat eggs or dairy—work with a nutritionist to ensure you are eating the right mix of whole foods. And no one should take any nutritional supplements other than a quality prenatal vitamin and pharmaceutical-grade fish oil during pregnancy without first discussing the pros and cons with a health care practitioner. (See Appendix E.)

Throughout the rest of this chapter, you'll discover what to eat—and what not to eat—during pregnancy.

Can I Diet While Pregnant?

No. A woman who is thinking about having a baby should try to achieve her ideal weight long before she conceives. (At least 2,200 calories a day are needed to support the growth of the developing fetus, so pregnancy is not the time for dieting.)

Being overweight during pregnancy is a problem because it increases the risk of complications, such as high blood pressure and gestational diabetes.

Being underweight isn't healthy either. Women who are more than 15 percent under normal weight are at risk of complications during pregnancy and childbirth.

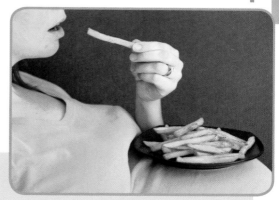

Food Cravings During Pregnancy

About two-thirds of women experience food cravings during pregnancy. It's usually fine to indulge your craving if it provides essential nutrients, but if your craving is for an unhealthy food or persists to the point that it prevents you from getting the other essential nutrients your baby needs, you need to take steps to create more balance in your daily diet and make sure that you take your prenatal vitamin.

Some women feel strong urges to eat nonfood items such as ice, laundry starch, dirt, clay, chalk, ashes, or paint chips when they are pregnant. This is known as pica, and it may be associated with anemia. These nonfood cravings can be harmful to both you and your baby, so it is very important that you resist them and tell your health care provider about them immediately.

If you have any cravings that interfere with your ability to eat balanced meals and gain weight properly, ask your obstetrician for advice. Registered dietitians—the nutrition experts—are also able to help you maintian good nutrition throughout your pregnancy.

What to Eat During Pregnancy

AS WAS MENTIONED ON the previous pages, healthy food choices during pregnancy are very important for your baby's growth and development. Although nausea, heartburn, and other digestive difficulties during pregnancy can interfere with your nutritional goals, try to eat a balanced diet and take your prenatal vitamins. Here are some additional recommendations to keep you and your baby healthy.

Dr. Colbert Approved

"Eat This" While Pregnant

- **Variety:** It's important to eat a wide variety of foods to ensure that you are getting all the nutrients you need. I recommend five or more servings of whole grains, two to four servings of fruit, three or more servings of vegetables, three or four servings of low-fat dairy products, and three servings of lean protein sources, organic preferred (meat, poultry, fish, eggs, or nuts). Use sugars sparingly or not at all, and choose healthy fats such as avocados, nuts, seeds, and extra-virgin olive oil.

- **Fiber:** Choose foods that are naturally high in fiber, such as fruits and vegetables (especially beans) or foods that have been enriched with extra fiber, such as high-fiber breads and cereals.

- **Folic acid:** Take your prenatal vitamin, which contains folic acid, but also consider eating a serving of foods rich in folic acid every day. Good sources include dark green leafy vegetables (spinach, kale, turnip greens, endive, broccoli), and legumes (lima beans, black beans, black-eyed peas, and chickpeas). The RDA during pregnancy is 0.6 mg a day.

- **Iron:** Consider eating a couple of iron-rich foods daily (the RDA for iron during pregnancy is 27 mg per day). Iron-containing foods include spinach, alfalfa, watercress, cabbage, parsley, currants and raisins, blackberries, and eggs fuel the rapidly expanding blood volume needed to supply the fetus. Fresh fruits that contain vitamin C will enhance your iron absorption.

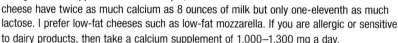

- **Calcium:** Eat or drink at least four servings of low-fat or skim milk dairy products or calcium-rich foods every day (to get the 1,000–1,300 mg of calcium you need during pregnancy). Unlike maternal iron stores, which are relatively small, maternal calcium stores are large. Adequate dietary calcium intake is easy for you to achieve if you consume dairy products (1 quart of milk contains 1,200 mg of calcium). If you must avoid dairy products because of lactose intolerance, you can get the calcium you need by substituting low-fat cheese for milk or taking calcium supplements. For example, 2 ounces of Swiss cheese have twice as much calcium as 8 ounces of milk but only one-eleventh as much lactose. I prefer low-fat cheeses such as low-fat mozzarella. If you are allergic or sensitive to dairy products, then take a calcium supplement of 1,000–1,300 mg a day.

- **Vitamin D:** Daily supplementation with 2,000 IUs of vitamin D should be considered for complete vegetarians and for persons who avoid sunlight. The RDA of vitamin D during pregnancy has been set at 200 IU a day. (See page 40.)

- **B-complex vitamins**: Except for vitamin B_{12}, the other B vitamins—thiamine, riboflavin, niacin, B_5 and B_6—are plentiful in a diet that includes a mix of vegetables, dairy products, and whole grains. Foods of animal origin are also good sources of all the Bs (including vitamin B_{12}). Getting enough vitamin B_{12} may be particularly problematic for vegetarians; this B vitamin is essential for the baby's developing blood supply and nervous system. Prenatal vitamin formulations also provide a healthy and balanced dose of the B complex vitamins.

- **Vitamin A:** At least 800 RE (retinol equivalent, used for quantifying the vitamin A value of sources of vitamin A) from foods such as carrots, pumpkins, sweet potatoes, spinach, winter squash, turnip greens, beet greens, apricots, and cantaloupe are recommended. This nutrient is essential for growth and development of skin, eyes, and the tissues lining the respiratory, intestinal, and urinary tracts. High doses of vitamin A (not beta-carotene) may cause birth defects and should be avoided (take no more than 5,000 IU of vitamin A a day).

- **Vitamin C:** This is another example of moderation is good, but excessive amounts are potentially dangerous." Eight ounces of orange juice deliver the 60 mg required for the nonpregnant woman, so it's easy to drink a bit more or eat more broccoli, red or green pepper, or strawberries for the additional 10 mg required in pregnancy. Most prenatal vitamins also contain some vitamin C. Megadoses of vitamin C, however, can possibly cause scurvy—a severe vitamin C deficiency disease—in the newborn, because once outside the mother's body, the large doses of C are abruptly cut off.

What to Avoid During Pregnancy

PREGNANCY OFTEN CREATES A greater understanding of the importance of lifestyle choices for expecting mothers and fathers. The dynamic of a developing fetus highlights, in a recognizable way, the significance of your lifestyle choices far more dramatically than when you think about the effects of such choices on yourself or other adults. Take advantage of this unique season of added awareness to make lifestyle changes that can help ensure your baby's healthy development and, if made permanent, can improve your long-term health as well.

Since alcohol, smoking, drugs (whether prescribed or illicit), and some nutritional supplements can harm the egg, sperm, or developing fetus, especially in the critical early days of gestation, couples should take exceptional care if they are thinking of having a baby. Here are some specifics on what to avoid before and during pregnancy.

Don't "Eat This" (or Drink This) While Pregnant

- Avoid alcohol during pregnancy, especially during the first few weeks when the most damaging effects of alcohol take place. Alcohol has been linked to premature delivery, birth defects, and low-birth-weight babies. Additionally, fetal alcohol syndrome (FAS) has been identified in children born to women who drink alcohol during their pregnancies.[2] The symptoms of FAS include growth retardation and developmental delays.

- Smoking during pregnancy increases the risk of complications, premature delivery, low-birth-weight babies (which is a leading cause of infant deaths), stillbirth, and SIDS (sudden infant death syndrome). In addition, babies born to women who smoke during pregnancy have reduced lung function.[3]

- It's wise to cut back on foods that have drug-like effects. Caffeine, for example, is a diuretic and contains potentially dangerous alkaloids; recommended limits on coffee range from one to three cups a day. Keep in mind a standard coffee cup is 6 ounces.

- Artificial sweeteners should be avoided during pregnancy, especially aspartame. Women who are heavy drinkers of diet soda, for example, should consider switching to a beverage like tea or water without artificial sweeteners and containing no phenylalanine or aspartic acid, which can reach the fetus.

- Do not eat shark, swordfish, king mackerel, or tilefish (also called white snapper), because they contain high levels of mercury. The American College of Obstetricians and Gynecologists recommends pregnant women limit fish to two 6-ounce servings a week.

- Avoid raw fish, especially shellfish like oysters and clams.

- Limit sugar since it's associated with excessive weight gain during pregnancy.

Herbs and Drugs to Avoid

Discuss with your physician the necessity of taking any drugs that you are currently prescribed. The following drugs and herbs are known to cause harm during pregnancy:

- Retin A (isotretinoin), Accutane, and high doses of vitamin A can cause birth defects. Accutane, a derivative of vitamin A used to treat acne, can cause serious birth defects.

- Certain anticonvulsants

- Iodine-containing drugs

- High doses of aspirin

- Certain high blood pressure medications known as angiotensin-converting enzyme (ACE) inhibitors

- Certain antibiotics, such as tetracycline, streptomycin, gentamicin, and kanamycin

- Lithium

- Strong bitter herbs, such as feverfew, tansy, goldenseal, mugwort, and barberry

- Herbs that contain alkaloids, including goldenseal, bloodroot, broom, mandrake, and barberry

- Any herb oil

- Laxative herbs, including senna and cascara

- Peruvian bark, poke, cotton root, and male fern

- Be aware that cocaine diminishes blood supply to the uterus and can cause neurologic damage and retard the baby's growth.

BREAST-FEEDING

THE BENEFITS OF BREAST-FEEDING

THE BENEFITS OF BREAST-FEEDING are numerous for both mom and baby. The more breast milk a baby gets, the better; and the benefits of nursing are greater for babies nursed for a year or more than for babies nursed only a few weeks or months. Partial breast-feeding—along with formula—protects babies against disease, but exclusive breast-feeding does so even better.

There is some evidence that breast-feeding reduces the risk of SIDS (sudden infant death syndrome). Bottle-fed American infants are fourteen times more likely to be hospitalized than breast-fed infants.[1]

The benefits of nursing extend well beyond the actual nursing period, protecting babies against diseases like type 1 diabetes, lymphoma, allergies, asthma, and Crohn's disease during childhood and potentially protecting them against these and other illnesses in adulthood.[2] A breast-fed infant has better immunity against childhood diseases, especially respiratory diseases, gastrointestinal infections, and ear infections. Breast milk strengthens a baby's immune system in responding to any challenge.

Because of the superior bioavailability of the nutrients in human milk, your baby will absorb and utilize more of the nutrients in food than a formula-fed child. Breast milk is free, always sanitized, always warm, and matched to the day-to-day, hour-to-hour needs of your baby.

I will discuss and compare breastmilk and infant formulas in the next chapter. See pages 47–52 for my formula recommendations.

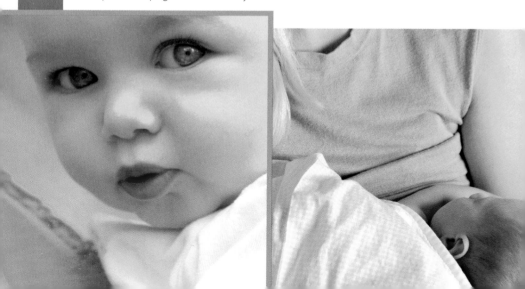

Your Child's Lifelong Relationship With Food Starts Now

Your child's appetite—his or her like and dislike of certain foods—is forming from the very first feeding. And children's nutrition in the first five years determines the quality of the rest of their lives. Parents' greatest challenge is to find, prepare, and feed nutritious whole food to their children consistently. Parents must teach by example, offering nutritious food—whole food, the closest to nature.

Interaction From Dad

Dads can feel left out in nourishing their babies with moms exclusively breast-feeding. Lactation consultants advise that moms can begin pumping and providing breast milk for dads to bottle-feed babies at six weeks. For earlier dad involvement, try skin-to-skin therapy—infant massage—which nourishes the baby emotionally and mentally.

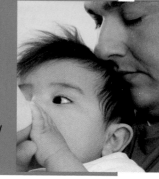

For Those Who Choose Not to Nurse

There are times when a mother feels she can't give her baby her best if she is breast-feeding and hating it or not making enough milk. My goal is not to make you feel guilty or judged—or to make you fear for your child's health—if you've tried your best at breast-feeding but formula was the right choice for you. I still say the more breast milk you can feed your baby, the better. But you can rest easy that formula is better now than it has ever been.

Breast-Feeding Benefits Moms Too

For you as the mother, there are many benefits to exclusive breast-feeding for at least six months.

1. Your fertility is reduced, with the chances of conceiving again during the period of breast-feeding reduced to about 2 percent. A non-nursing mother can be fertile again within fifty days of giving birth.

2. Your long-term risk of breast cancer and osteoporosis fall.

3. Your bonding with your baby is improved.

4. Hormonal changes linked with lactation will aid you in making good mothering choices and weathering the inevitable storms that come with having a new baby.

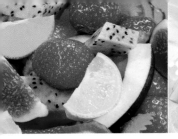
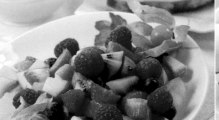
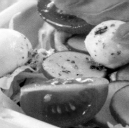

Make Sure You and Your Baby Are Getting the Right Nutrients

WHEN YOU'RE BREAST-FEEDING, IT'S important to get the needed vitamins and minerals into your body and your baby's body via carefully chosen nutrient-dense foods. A good prenatal multivitamin-mineral and a pharmaceutical-grade fish oil supplement are smart insurance against deficiencies, but remember that they are supplements designed to support a healthy diet—not the other way around.

Healthy foods should always be your primary source of vitamins and minerals because these nutrients are designed to work in teams in the context of whole foods. A piece of spinach is a synergetic dance of vitamins, minerals, antioxidants, phytonutrients, fiber, fatty acids, proteins, water, accessory nutrients, and a lot of things we haven't even discovered yet. A vitamin made from lab-created, isolated vitamins and minerals doesn't match up, any more than baby formula matches up with the fresh milk in a lactating woman's breasts.

Unfortunately, calorie-dense, highly processed foods made from refined sugar, flour, corn, and oil are main staples of our modern diet. These foods give us plenty of energy—much of which ends up stored as fat—but they don't offer high concentrations of the micronutrients we require. For your baby's health while breast-feeding, it's much better to avoid these foods and instead turn to fresh whole foods supported by nutritional supplements.

Antioxidant Protection From Day One

The total antioxidant capacity of breast milk is higher in moms who consume more antioxidants in food and as supplements. Take in a wide variety of antioxidant-rich foods and supplements like leafy green vegetables, green tea, berries, citrus fruits, and red grapes; don't rely on high-dose supplements of single antioxidants like C or E.

The Link Between Mindful Eating and Nursing

Eating with *mindfulness* (being present in the moment when eating) may actually affect the way food is metabolized, which ultimately affects health and well-being. A breast-feeding mom with negative feelings tends to consume more processed foods and is less likely to eat fresh whole food. She tends to pay less attention to the sensory and spiritual aspects of eating. Food-related thoughts are more likely to focus on self-judgment and feeling bad.

So it's important to be aware of your emotions not only while you're nursing your baby but also when you're eating your own meals. Maternal eating styles have a profound influence on mother-baby relationship building and the successfulness of the breast-feeding experience.

Storing Breast Milk Reduces Vitamin C Content

For moms who pump and store breast milk: keep in mind that after twenty-four hours in the refrigerator, human milk has lost, on average, a third of its vitamin C. A month in the freezer has the same effect. The range of vitamin C loss varies between 6 and 76 percent in the fridge and 3 to 100 percent in the freezer.

Avoid storing milk for more than a few hours in the fridge if you want to ensure optimal nutritional value. If you won't be using it within a few hours, freeze it and use it within a week or two. If you have to use milk stored for long periods, consider adding 20 to 40 mg of powdered vitamin C in the ascorbate form (it's buffered so that it is not acidic; most vitamin C supplements are in the form of ascorbic acid) to the bottle before feeding.

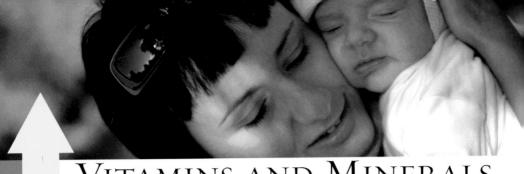

VITAMINS AND MINERALS FOR NURSING MOMS

VITAMINS AND MINERALS—YOU NEED them—you've used a lot of your body's nutrient stores to form a baby—to maintain growth, development, immunity, and day-to-day physiological function. Continue to take your prenatal vitamin while breastfeeding. (See Appendix E.) Here's a quick list of vitamins important during breast-feeding.

- **Vitamin B_{12}** creates and maintains DNA and RNA, the genetic templates from which our cells are made. A growing baby's body is making new cells rapidly. If B_{12} is not available in adequate supply, growth and development suffer. Who is at greatest risk of deficiency? Vegans who avoid all animal products, including meat and eggs. They should take special care to take a B_{12} supplement, especially while nursing, as well as continue to take their prenatal vitamin.

- **Folic acid/folate** plays a major role in producing and maintaining new cells. Eat plenty of green vegetables, whole grains, and beans.

- **Vitamin B_6** plays an integral role in the functioning of the nervous and immune systems. The risk of B_6 deficiency is higher in babies who are exclusively breast-fed beyond six months of age. If your breast-fed baby shows little or no interest in solid foods, you can insure adequate amounts of B_6 go into your breast milk by eating foods rich in B_6, plus take a quality multivitamin or prenatal vitamin.

- **Vitamin D** is made in the skin from the combination of cholesterol and ultraviolet rays from the sun. An exclusively breast-fed child who is kept completely out of the sun can become deficient in vitamin D. But adequate amounts of vitamin D for a nursing baby can be achieved without sup-plements if both nursing mom and baby get fifteen to twenty minutes of sunshine two or three days a week. If a nursing mom gets adequate sunlight, then baby will typically get adequate amounts of vitamin D in the breast milk.

- **Vitamin C** is important for good immune system function. Any nursing mother who can't eat foods rich in vitamin C on a daily basis should supplement with this nutrient, plus take a prenatal vitamin.

Sources of Vitamins and Antioxidants

Vitamin	RDA	Good Food Source	Supplements
B_{12}	2.4 mcg	Poultry, fish, beef, eggs	Present in prenatal vitamin or quality multivitamin (See Appendix E)
Folic acid	600 mcg (if pregnant) 500 mcg (if nursing)	Green vegetables, whole grains, beans	Available in a quality prenatal vitamin
B_6	2.0 mg	Fish, meat, nuts, cereals, whole grains	25–50 mg
D	200 IU	Fish, egg yolks, fortified dairy	Take at least 200 IU of vitamin D_3 a day; tolerable upper limits are 2,000 IU a day. I personally recommend 2,000 IU and having a 25OHD3 level blood test.
C	80 mg (if pregnant)	Citrus fruits, strawberries, tomatoes, sweet red peppers, broccoli	100 mg/day
A	2,567 IU (if pregnant)	Fortified breakfast cereals, eggs, butter, milk	3,000 IU retinol or 5,000 IU vitamin A with half as beta-carotene; also present in prenatal vitamin or quality multivitamin
Carotenes	None	Yams, carrots, cantaloupe, kale, spinach	None needed; best to get from diet; can get some to fulfill needs of vitamin A
K	65 mcg	Leafy greens, dairy products	RDA can usually be found in a good multivitamin or prenatal vitamin

Sources of Minerals

Mineral	RDA	Good Food Source	Supplements
Iron	30 mg	Kelp, wheat bran, pumpkin seeds, almonds, millet, lean beef, poultry, fish, deep green leafy vegetables, pork, eggs	Consult with your practitioner to see if iron is needed and how much you should take
Calcium	1,000–1,300 mg	Dairy products, green leafy vegetables, sardines (with bones), tofu, broccoli, calcium-fortified orange juice	1,000–1,500 mg a day in divided doses
Selenium	60 mcg (if pregnant) 70 mcg (if nursing)	Beef, turkey, seafood, wheat germ, Brazil nuts, barley, red chard, brown rice	70–100 mcg
Iodine	220 mcg	Seafood, seaweed	150 mcg

THE PROPER CARE AND FEEDING OF YOUR BABY AND TODDLER

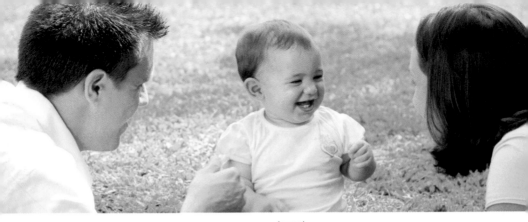

MAKING THE TRANSITION FROM BREAST TO BOTTLE

YOUR REASONS FOR DECIDING to bottle-feed will have a profound effect on how quickly and efficiently the transition from breast to bottle will take place. When deciding how to feed your baby, the importance of teaming up with a lactation consultant cannot be overstated.

Remember, once you have made the decision to bottle-feed, you must see your family as a group functioning to achieve and sustain harmony, balance, and ultimately well-being in your baby's life.

Making a Smooth Transition

Look for a lactation consultant who practices mind-body medicine with parents and baby during this transition period. You'll want a consultant who helps you with stress management and relaxation to help you achieve the appropriate mind-set. This is more important than you might think, because your baby can sense your emotions; rather than stress, you want him to sense your gentle determination that he will learn this new way to obtain nourishment. Once your baby receives this powerful message coming from very confident parents, the transition to bottle comes down successfully and in short order.

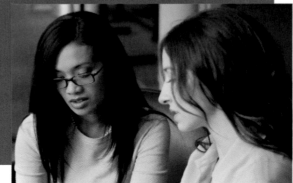

A Word From Dr. Cannizzaro:
FAQs About Bottle-Feeding

Here are answers to some questions I am asked when moms are switching to bottle-feeding. Hopefully these will provide you with some guidelines for the transition.

- **How much should I feed my baby?** Expect a newborn up to two months old to take 1–2 ounces each feeding; a two- to six-month-old should take 3–4 ounces each feeding; a six- to twelve-month-old should take 4–6 ounces each feeding and 8 ounces each feeding thereafter.

- **How often will my baby eat?** Because formula is more filling than breast milk, a formula-fed baby will probably be on a four-hour schedule around the clock until he or she sleeps through the night. I advise moms to let their babies communicate with them when they are hungry, and they'll get on their own schedule naturally.

- **How do I know if there is adequate flow?** To check for adequate milk flow, turn filled bottle upside down. Liquid should come out at one drop per second.

- **How do I know if my baby is full?** When your baby "spits the nipple out," don't try to have him finish any remaining formula. A baby's stomach is only about as big as her fist, and she won't drain a full bottle every time. If she eats too much, her tiny stomach will send some of it back out. Small frequent feedings are better than fewer feedings with long intervals between. Heed your baby's hunger signals early, and don't press her to drink past the point when she seems satiated.

- **What if my baby falls asleep while eating?** Your baby might fall asleep while drinking from a bottle. If this happens, once her deeper drinking sucks give way to little fluttery sucks, take the bottle out and replace it with a pacifier to prevent overfeeding.

- **Are there any signs that my baby is not getting enough nutrition from bottle-feeding?** Signs of dehydration or inadequate formula consumption include slow weight gain, fewer than six to eight wet diapers per day, persistent crying, depressed fontanel (soft spot on crown of the head), or skin that looks loose or wrinkly.

- **Can a baby be left alone with his bottle?** Never prop a bottle or put your baby to bed with a bottle in his mouth. Feeding, whether from a bottle or breast, should be a time for closeness and cuddling. If you can, hold your baby skin-to-skin while bottle-feeding. See page 46 for more transition tips.

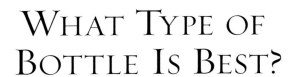

WHAT TYPE OF BOTTLE IS BEST?

SOME MOMS CHOOSE TO breast-feed but cannot always be there in person to feed their child. Whether you are providing breast milk or infant formula via the bottle, there are some things to keep in mind when choosing which bottles to offer your child.

Bottles made from polycarbonate plastic are convenient and easy to find, but research has shown that hormone-disrupting chemicals, specifically bisphenol A (BPA), readily migrate out into the liquid inside the bottle[1]. If polycarbonate is used, the older the bottles, the more BPA they'll shed. This is why I recommend that you find alternatives to these types of bottles. Here's what the Children's Health Environmental Coalition has to say about safe baby bottles:

- Glass bottles are making a comeback. Evenflow is the company that sells them. The only risk with glass bottles is cracking or chipping. Watch for cracks and chips, and discard immediately if found.

- Polyethylene or polypropylenes do not leak any hormone disrupters. Medela, Evenflow, and Gerber make these types of bottles. Soft plastic liners are another option. No research thus far demonstrates that these liners release toxic chemicals, but they have been known to cause choking accidents.

Choosing a Nipple

If a baby is both bottle- and breast-feeding, choose a nipple that has a wide base to mimic the sensation of mom's breast. Using a standard longer nipple can cause nipple confusion and create a lazy nurser who only wants to take the whole nipple and most of the areola. Here are a few more tips:

- Rubber nipples may shed nitrosamines, a carcinogenic chemical. Choose bottle nipples and pacifiers made from natural latex or silicone.
- There is no conclusive evidence that so-called "orthodontic nipples" are superior to others.
- Boil nipples for five minutes before first using them.
- If any cracks or tears appear, toss the nipple in the trash to avoid a choking hazard.

More Transition Tips

- Introduce the bottle before you need to. Plan to start offering the bottle several weeks before the transition needs to be completed.

- Gradual change, such as substituting the bottle at one feeding every three to five days to start, is best. Eventually work your way up to substituting the bottle for one feeding a day. A gradual switch like this will help reduce your baby's stress over the change while at the same time helping you avoid engorgement as your body adapts to less demand for breast milk.

- If you're offering breast milk in the bottle rather than formula, have dad or another caregiver offer bottles. This gives dad a chance to bond while also helping your baby adapt her expectations at feeding time.

- Don't try weaning if your baby is cutting a tooth. The pain and discomfort she's feeling will give her enough to deal with already; save feeding transitions for another day.

- Skip the bottle and go straight to a cup if your child is more than twelve months old.

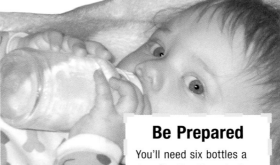

Be Prepared

You'll need six bottles a day. Sterilize them in the dishwasher, or hand wash in hot soapy water, rinse, place in pan, or boil for ten minutes.

Defrosting Frozen Bottles

Never defrost a bottle of frozen breast milk in the microwave. Defrost frozen bottles by placing them on the counter for about thirty minutes or by placing them in the refrigerator for a few hours before your baby needs to be fed. Then warm them according to the information about heating bottles on this page.

Heating Bottles

Never heat bottles in a microwave. Instead, use a bottle warmer, or hold it under warm running tapwater, or boil a cup of water in the microwave and then set the bottle in the cup of hot water on the counter for a minute or two.

Is Baby Formula OK?

ALL BABY FORMULAS SOLD in stores or given out in hospitals or doctors' offices have been prepared according to strict FDA guidelines. The following types of formula are available:

- Cow's milk-based formula: proteins come from nonfat milk and whey protein concentrate; fats from palm, safflower, sunflower, corn, coconut, soybean oils; carbohydrates from lactose (milk sugars), maltodextrin, corn syrup

- Soy formula: proteins come from soy protein isolate; fats from palm, safflower, sunflower, corn, coconut, soy oils; carbohydrates from corn syrup solids, sucrose (sugar)

- Lactose-free formula (contains no milk sugar, but does contain milk proteins, which may be allergenic to some babies): proteins from whey, casein (milk proteins), nonfat milk with milk sugars removed; fats from palm, soy, coconut, sunflower oils; sugars from corn syrup, sucrose (sugar)

- Premature formulas (available in soy- and milk-based forms)

- Formulas supplemented with DHA and ARA (available in all of the above): DHA and ARA are typically derived from fish oils, or algae.

- Elemental (hypoallergenic) formula: protein from hydrolyzed (predigested) casein; fats from safflower, coconut, soy oils; sweetened with corn syrup, dextrose, or modified corn or tapioca starch. One such formula, Pregestimil, gets its fat from medium-chain triglycerides, a factory-made fat.

- Follow-up formulas are also available. They are designed for babies aged four to six months and older and contain a slightly different balance of nutrients, with more calcium, protein, and iron than regular baby formulas. As long as your baby is eating solid foods with gusto by six months, the extra nutrients are probably not necessary.

Watch for Corn Syrup

Many follow-up formulas are sweetened with corn syrup—the same sugars used to sweeten most sodas. In order to avoid whetting your baby's tastes to favor sweetness, avoid those made with corn syrup if at all possible.

A baby who turns his nose up at solids may be a good candidate for a follow-up formula, but his nutritional needs can probably be filled with slightly increased intake of standard formula plus some solid foods that contain calcium and iron.

Are organic formulas better?

Organic formulas are now available, but they are so new that no one knows whether organic makes a difference; just because an infant formula is given the "organic" label doesn't necessarily mean that it is healthy.

For example, a recent article in the *New York Times* revealed that the organic version of Similac infant formula is sweetened with cane sugar (sucrose) and is much sweeter than other infant formulas.[2] While all infant formulas have some added sugars to aid in the digestion of proteins, organic products usually use sugars like organic lactose, which is presumably a better match for what's found in breast milk and doesn't have the sweetness of sucrose.

Any substance that is generally recognized as safe may be used in infant formula in the United States. For now, that means that sugar can be used in baby formula in the States, and there is absolutely no upper limit to the amount of sugar that can be dumped into it. Europe, on the other hand, in light of the childhood obesity epidemic, has banned all sucrose from baby formula products beginning in 2009.

According to the *New York Times* article, Dr. Benjamin Caballero, director of the Johns Hopkins Bloomberg School of Public Health, also doesn't think sucrose belongs in infant formula. Dr. Caballero believes that feeding children sweet things encourages them to eat more. He explains that babies and children generally prefer sweeter foods and will eat more of them than foods that aren't as sweet.[3]

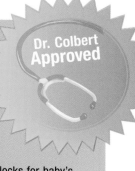

DHA and ARA Formulas

Dr. Colbert Approved

I recommend any brand that adds DHA (docosahexaenoic acid) and ARA (arachidonic acid) to its formulas. These fats in formula are building blocks for baby's nervous system and visual development.

Soy Formulas

Soy formulas have a lengthy history of apparently safe use, but there are potential downsides. For instance, consumption of soy has been related to thryroid problems, endocrine disruption, asthma, and reproductive disorders, and the genistein in soy has been shown to cause cancer in rats. More research needs to be done before we make the final call on soy, but until then, these concerns are enough for me to say that soy is not my first choice. If you do choose soy formula, it should be used exclusively for the first four to six months with solid foods (organic fruits and vegetables) being added at that time.

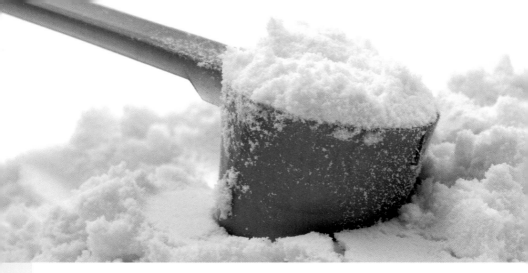

ENHANCING COMMERCIAL BABY FORMULA

BEFORE YOU MAKE A final decision on whether to use commercial baby formula or not, I would like to make you aware of a few steps you can take to make store-bought formulas just a little more nutritionally sound and "alive."

- Formula companies have started adding prebiotics and probiotics to formulas. Prebiotics are non-digestible food ingredients such as fructo-oligosaccharides (FOS), a type of carbohydrate that is a favorite food for the beneficial bacteria and that promotes their growth and activity. Probiotics are products or supplements that contain live, active beneficial bacterial cultures. Beneficial bacteria called lacto bacilli (acidophilus and bifidus) inhibit the growth of bad bacteria in the gastrointestinal tract and enhance immunity.

  If you purchase a formula that does not come with probiotics already added, you can add them yourself. I recommend a brand of probiotics made especially for infants. (See Appendix E.) Add the recommended amount to your baby's bottle, or dust the recommended amount on the nipple of the bottle or pacifier once a day. Keep probiotics stored in the refrigerator.

- To enhance the development of baby's immune system, I recommend the addition of a concentrated whole-food micronutrient powder to the formula. (See Appendix E.) The contents of one capsule can be dissolved in 1 ounce of formula and fed to your baby immediately.

- Formulas can also be supplemented with soft-cooked organic egg yolk. Use DHA-rich eggs, which are now widely available. Boil the egg for three and a half minutes. Remove the egg white, which is allergenic to babies less than one year old. Mix into formula, one yolk per 35 ounces of formula. Cod liver oil can be added to formula, ½ teaspoon per 35 ounces; make sure this formula is not DHA fortified.

- Some sources recommend adding cod liver oil to formulas as a source of natural DHA. If you do so, choose a formula without added DHA. Use only ½ teaspoon per 35-ounce batch, and add it along with the egg yolk. Never use soy milk, rice milk, carrot juice, or almond milk as a replacement for formula or breast milk.

- Lastly, lactose intolerance is not nearly as common in children as it is widely believed to be. It runs counter to common sense that an infant would be allergic to the carbohydrate that is specifically designed to feed human babies. Lactose intolerance and milk allergy are often confused. They are quite different and unrelated; they don't even involve the same body system. Lactose intolerance is a digestive issue; milk allergy is an immune system problem. Lactose intolerance is the result of a lack of the enzyme lactase, the enzyme that breaks lactose down in the digestive tract. This can be a temporary problem just following an intestinal infection. A lactose-free formula can be used for a brief time. Formulas that don't supply sugar as lactose will usually contain corn syrup or maltodextrin—more refined sugars that are not optimal for growing babies. Allergy to cow milk protein is very common, and if you switch to a soy-based formula, keep in mind that 30 to 50 percent of babies who are allergic to milk proteins are often allergic to soy.

Problems Digesting Iron-Fortified Formulas

Most formulas are fortified with iron. A nursing infant absorbs 100 percent of the iron in mother's milk, but the iron-fortified formula is much more poorly absorbed. This can lead to constipation. There are low-iron formulas, but then there's the issue of the baby possibly not getting adequate iron. Babies have enough iron stored up from being inside mom's body to last four months of life as long as mom's iron levels were adequate during pregnancy. Babies who don't tolerate iron-fortified formulas can be given low-iron formulas to start with and then an iron supplement beginning at four months or age.

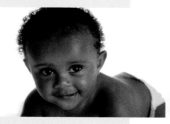

ALTERNATIVES TO COMMERCIAL BABY FORMULA

I GENERALLY DISCOURAGE THE practice of making your own baby formula because it's difficult to know whether it is meeting the nutritional needs of the infant. Today's formulas are the best they've ever been. They are not as good as breast milk and aren't even close. But they come in second place to breast milk, hands down.

I strongly recommend any mom with the intention of substituting anything for breast milk to work closely with a lactation consultant, an integrative nutritionist, and also a compounding pharmacist who can help design a nutritionally balanced substitute to breast milk. The following breast milk substitutes are as good an approximation of breast milk as can be obtained without going to a commercial formula.

Here are two infant formulas to use if you cannot breast-feed your infant. Add commercial colostrum supplements soon after birth to more closely approximate natural breast milk. Note: Do not substitute honey for molasses, maple syrup, or cane sugar. Children under one year of age who eat honey are at risk for contracting botulism, a serious paralytic disease.

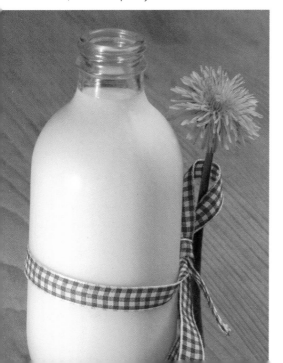

Goat's Milk Formula

- 2/3 qt. goat's milk (not low fat)
- 1/2 qt. pure spring water
- 3 Tbsp. lactose
- After three months of age, add:
- 1/2 tsp. blackstrap molasses
- 1/2 tsp. brewer's yeast

Wright-Lauffer Formula

- 1 qt. soy milk
- 1 cup carrot juice
- 1/4 tsp. barley greens
- 1/4 tsp. nutritional yeast
- 200 IU vitamin D
- 100 mg. ascorbate (vitamin C) powder
- 1 Tbsp. safflower oil (pure, expeller-pressed)
- 3 Tbsp. pure maple syrup or lactose

Omega-3 Oils

Some homemade formula recipes call for fish or flaxseed oil as an omega-3 source or for cod liver oil. I would not recommend you to supplement infant formulas that do not contain extra DHA (docosahexaenoic acid) or ARA (arachidonic acid) with fish oil or flaxseed oil alone because neither of these oils contains a source of ARA. A relative dearth of ARA compared to DHA and EPA (eicosapentaenoic acid) can slow a baby's growth. Homemade formula supplementation recipes may call for the addition of a soft-cooked egg yolk to contribute this fat.

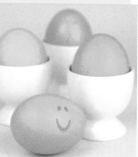

Substituting With Goat's Milk

Goat's milk can be a good replacement for breast feeding for the first ten to twelve months. It should be diluted (3 parts goat's milk to 1 part water). Be sure it is supplemented with folic acid and iron as recommended by your pediatrician. Goat's milk is believed to be more easily digestible and less allergenic than cow's milk.

Different fat: Unlike cow's milk, goat's milk does not contain agglutinin. As a result, the fat globules in goat's milk do not cluster together, making them easier to digest. Goat's milk contains more of the essential fatty acids linoleic and arachidonic than cow's milk, in addition to a higher proportion of short-chain and medium-chain fatty acids; these are easier for intestinal enzymes to digest.

Different protein: Goat milk protein forms a softer curd (the term given to the protein clumps that are formed by the action of your stomach acid), which makes the protein more easily and rapidly digestible. Less reflux is seen in infants on goat's milk compared to cow's milk. Goat's milk may also have advantages when it comes to allergies. It contains only trace amounts of an allergenic casein protein alpha that is found in cow's milk. Goat milk casein is more similar to human milk. Mothers frequently describe their children tolerating goat's milk better than cow's milk.

EATING FOR THE FIRST YEAR

NEW PARENTS OFTEN WONDER how they will know their baby is ready for solid foods. As a general rule, a baby who is ready for solids will start grabbing at your food and watching intently the path your fork full of food takes from your plate to your mouth. However, it's important not to rush into trying too many different solids too soon. There are three concepts to keep in mind.

1. **Make your little one a "whole-foods baby"!** Avoid processed and refined foods as much as possible, including many brands of commercial baby food; some are lacking nutrients and have added "undesirables." It is always best to make your own baby food from organic, whole foods. (You can freeze it in one-serving sizes for later use.) Better-quality, additive-free, prepared brands of baby food, like Earth's Best, do exist, but it is still better to make your own baby food to be assured of the quality. Plus, making baby food puts you as a parent on the right track for home food preparation for the years to come.

2. **Go slowly and be observant.** Every baby will have an individual response to different foods. Introduce new foods one at a time, and continue to feed that same food along with breast milk or formula for at least four days to rule out the possibility of a negative reaction. Signs of intolerance include redness around the mouth; abdominal bloating, gas, and distention; irritability, fussiness, overactivity, and awakening throughout the night; constipation and diarrhea; frequent regurgitation of foods; nasal and/or chest congestion; and red, chapped, or inflamed eczema-like skin rash.

3. **Respect the tiny, still-developing digestive system of your infant.** Babies have limited enzyme production, which is necessary for the digestion of foods. In fact, it takes up to twenty-eight months, just around the time when molar teeth are fully developed, for the big gun carbohydrate enzymes (namely amylase) to fully kick into gear. Foods like cereals, grains, and breads are very challenging for little ones to digest. Thus these foods should be the last to be introduced.

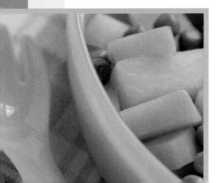

Babies do produce functional enzymes (pepsin and proteolytic enzymes) and digestive juices (hydrochloric acid in the stomach) that work on proteins and fats. This makes perfect sense since the milk from a healthy mother has 50-60 percent of its energy as fat, which is critical for growth, energy, and development. In addition, the cholesterol in human milk supplies an infant with close to six times the amount most adults consume from food. In some cultures, a new mother is encouraged to eat six to ten eggs a day and almost 10 ounces of chicken and pork for at least a month after birth. This fat-rich diet ensures her breast milk will contain adequate healthy fats.

Thus, a baby's earliest solid foods should be mostly animal foods since his digestive system, although immature, is better equipped to supply enzymes for digestion of fats and proteins rather than carbohydrates. This explains why current research is pointing to meat as being a nourishing early weaning food. See pages 55 and 60 for a list of which foods to introduce at which age.

Don't Start With Refined Carbs and Sugars

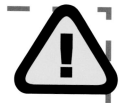

It's customary to give very young babies crackers, O-shaped cereal, bagels, or cookies, but there are several important reasons to avoid doing this.

- There is some evidence that introducing wheat too soon can promote oversensitivity to gluten in the baby's immature gut.

- The intense, almost sweet taste of these foods can spoil your baby's taste for more nutritious whole foods.

- Any refined carbohydrates or sugar can contribute to early tooth decay.

I recommend cereal introduction only after the baby has experienced a large variety of fruits and vege-tables. If you opt for commercially available cereal, use fortified instant rice cereal and mix it with some breast milk, plain live-culture yogurt, or formula. Offer at least two servings per day of puréed meat or fish, especially to the formula-fed baby.

A Word From Dr. Cannizzaro: Starting Solid Foods Too Soon Can Cause Allergies

Foods introduced too early can cause digestive troubles and increase the likelihood of allergies (particularly to those foods introduced). The baby's immature digestive system allows large particles of food to be absorbed. If these particles reach the bloodstream, the immune system may mount a response that leads to an allergic reaction. Six months is the typical age when solids should be introduced; however, there are a few exceptions.

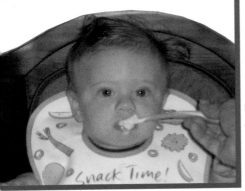

INTRODUCING FIRST FOODS

PARENTS OF FORMULA-FED BABIES may be able to start solids as early as four months, however, I feel it's best to start solid foods at six months of age to avoid food allergies. Postponing the introduction of solid foods and prolonging breast-feeding gives an infant's immune system enough time to adequately mature. A later introduction of solid foods, in particular peanuts, eggs, wheat, and fish, may reduce the incidence of allergies. In addition, children started on solid foods before the age of four months are more likely to experience chronic or recurrent episodes of eczema than children of the same age who were not introduced to solid foods.

When your child is ready to eat solid foods, usually after six months, you can give her a healthy start by devising a diet made up of fresh fruits and vegetables, legumes, and low-fat proteins such as chicken and fish. I recommend that you:

- Introduce foods one at a time (one new food every three days).
- Discontinue a food if allergy/sensitivity symptoms occur, such as rash, hyperactivity or lethargy, tantrums, runny nose, infections (especially ear), mucus in stools or diarrhea, or red cheeks.
- Provide a variety of foods, and don't give each food too often.

The most allergenic foods (dairy and wheat) should be introduced later. Be especially watchful for reactions with meats, corn, peanuts, and soy. Please refer to the chart on this page for my specific recommendations for introducing new foods during your child's first year of life.

Food Introduction Schedule					
Four Months (if formula-fed) **Six Months (if breast-fed)**		**Nine Months**		**Twelve Months**	
Applesauce	Cauliflower	Artichoke	Nectarine	Asparagus	Parsnips
Banana	Cherries(mashed)	Basmati rice	Oats	Avocado	Squash
Blackberries	Grapes (mashed)	Blueberries	Papaya	Barley	Swiss chard
Broccoli (cooked	Pears	(frozen helps	Potato (cooked	Blackstrap	Tofu
and blended)	Prunes	teething)	and mashed)	molasses	Yogurt
Carrot (cooked	Sprouts	Brown rice	Split peas	Goat's milk (fresh)	(if no reaction)
and mashed)	Yams	Cabbage	String beans		
		Lima beans			
		Millet			

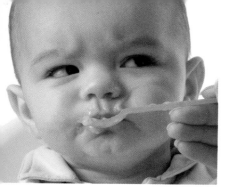

What If My Baby Doesn't Like New Foods?

Babies are neophobic (fearful of anything new), which is self-protective. If a food is initially rejected, the parent is advised to repeat offerings (sampling) until the process is complete, and the food will be consumed. For many obvious reasons food preparation for the baby at this age is pureed. For other practical reasons I recommend coverings for the wall and ceiling and the family dog for the floor.

Foods to Avoid

Do not give your child commercially prepared juice, which contains too much simple sugar and may ruin a child's appetite for the more nourishing food choices. Soy foods, margarine and shortening, and commercial dairy products (especially ultra-pasteurized) should also be avoided, as well as any products that are reduced fat or low fat.

How Much at Each Meal?

One food portion is equal to 1 tablespoon. Your baby will, most likely, only eat half of the small portion for the first few attempts with solids. Baby will show you how much he should eat. You can gradually increase the portion size once you have ruled out sensitivities/allergies to different foods. Be sure to rotate the food in the diet.

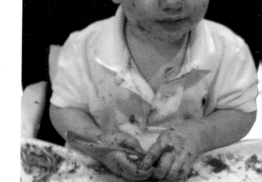

Eat on a Schedule

Children—even very young ones—thrive on routine. They like to know what to expect and what is expected of them. Sit down to eat on a regular schedule, even if baby doesn't actually eat. Allow him to touch, play with, smell, and otherwise manipulate his food. Don't stress about giving a specific amount of each food group each day. As long as breast milk or formula are part of the diet, his nutritional bases are probably covered.

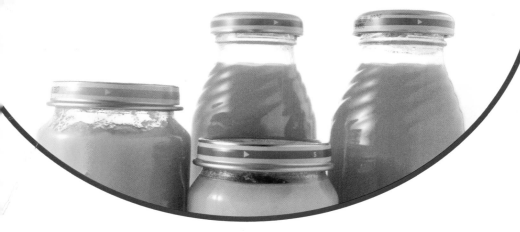

ALTERNATIVES TO COMMERCIAL BABY FOOD

IN PLACE OF COMMERCIAL baby food, try preparing the following foods for your child during the first year of life.

Homemade First-Year Foods	
Four Months (if formula-fed) Six Months (if breast-fed)	Give formula-fed babies some raw fruits that contain digestive enzymes, such as bananas, or other ripe fruit, thoroughly mashed. As a supplement to formula, a four-month-old baby can have freshly squeezed juice from organic fruits and vegetables to augment his consumption of living enzymes, which are naturally abundant in breast milk. Avoid citrus until nine months. Try puréeing fresh, raw apple and a lightly cooked carrot with a couple of tablespoons of fruit juice and a teaspoon of lemon juice. Mashed avocado, melon, mangoes, papaya, applesauce, peas, and cooked winter squash are all good first foods. (See chart on page 55 for more foods recommended at this age.) High-pectin fruits such as peaches, apricots, apples, pears, cherries, and berries should be cooked to break down the pectin, which can be very irritating to the digestive tract. Egg yolks, rich in choline, cholesterol, and other brain-nourishing substances, can be added to your baby's diet as early as four months, as long as baby takes it easily. (If baby reacts poorly to egg yolk at that age, discontinue and try again one month later.) Cholesterol is vital for the insulation of nerves in the brain and the entire central nervous system. It helps with fat digestion by increasing the formation of bile acids and is necessary for the production of many hormones. Since the brain is so dependent on cholesterol, it is especially vital during this time when brain growth is extremely rapid. Thus the best choice for baby is yolks from pasture-fed hens raised on flax meal, fish meal, or insects since they will contain higher levels of DHA. Why just the yolk? The white is the portion that most often causes allergic reactions, so wait to give egg whites until after your child turns one. Don't neglect to put a pinch of salt on the egg yolk. While many books warn against giving salt to babies, salt is actually critical for digestion as well as for brain development. Use unrefined salt to supply a variety of trace minerals.

	Homemade First-Year Foods
Six to Eight Months	As time goes by, move up in complexity with food and texture. At about six to eight months, vegetables may be introduced, one at a time so that any adverse reactions may be observed. Carrots, sweet potatoes, and beets are excellent first choices. All vegetables should be cooked (steamed preferably), mashed, and mixed with a liberal amount of fat, such as butter or coconut oil, to provide nutrients to aid in digestion. Early introduction to different tastes is always a good plan to prevent finickiness. Feed your little one a touch of buttermilk, yogurt, or kefir from time to time to familiarize them with the sour taste. Lacto-fermented roots, like sweet potato or taro, are another excellent food for babies to add at this time.
Eight Months	Baby can now consume a variety of foods and can handle a little bit of thickness and soft chunkiness in texture. Thicker foods include creamed vegetable soups, homemade stews, and dairy foods such as cottage cheese and custards. Hold off on grains until one year, with the possible exception of soaked and thoroughly cooked brown rice, which can be served earlier to babies who are very mature.
Twelve Months	Grains (like wheat), nuts, seeds, eggs, and fish should not be introduced until the infant is older than twelve months of age, especially if either parent has food sensitivities or allergies. This food category has the most potential for causing digestive disturbances or allergies. There has been a rise in peanut (legume) and nut allergies due to the trend of giving them to very young children. Babies do not produce the needed enzymes to handle cereal grains, especially gluten-containing grains like wheat, before the age of one year. Even then, it is common traditional practice to soak grains in water and a little yogurt or buttermilk for twenty-four hours. This process jump-starts the enzymatic activity in the food and begins breaking down some of the harder-to-digest components. The easiest grains to digest are those without gluten, like brown rice that has been soaked for at least twenty-four hours and cooked with plenty of water for a long time.

Don't Fear Fats!

Pediatric clinicians have known for some time that children fed low-fat and low-cholesterol diets fail to grow properly. Children need high levels of fat throughout growth and development. Milk and animal fats give energy and also help children build muscle and bone. In addition, the animal fats provide vitamins A and D necessary for protein and mineral assimilation, normal growth, and hormone production. Choose a variety of foods so your child gets a range of fats, but emphasize stable saturated fats, found in butter, meat, and coconut oils, and monounsaturated fats, found in avocados and olive oil.

Homemade Juices Are Best

The only juices I recommend are those made from fresh fruits or veggies (organic); leave the skin on most fruits and veggies. Choose phytonutrient-rich grape, pomegranate, or berries to juice. If juicing at home is not feasible for you, chunks of fruits and veggies can be placed in mesh (cheesecloth) bags and baby can chew and suck without biting off pieces that he/she can choke on. If you can't resist the convenience of jarred baby food, seek out organic versions.

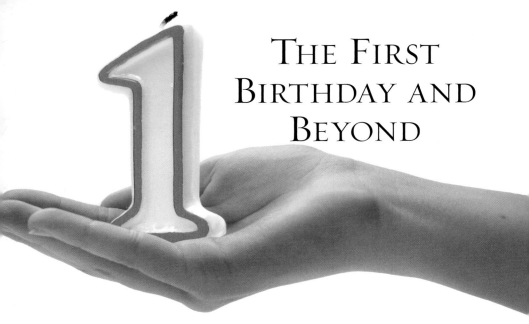

THE FIRST BIRTHDAY AND BEYOND

AS YOUR CHILD APPROACHES his or her first birthday, he or she is pulling up, holding on to anything in reach. Combine this skill with an incredible desire to learn all about his/ her environment, and you've got what I call a "toddler in training."

By twelve months, toddlers can and will eat just about everything parents eat, but they have gone from gaining 2 pounds a month to 2 pounds a year, and they can become "picky." Since they don't want increased bulk, small portions of a large variety of foods at one meal is the key. Let them graze; it's their physiology. If they are given foods that are chemically laden, calorically dense, energy rich, but nutrient poor, a false sense of fullness sets in, and they begin to refuse the natural foods they need.

Along with appetite development, bowel habits are given major emphasis at our continuity visits. What should stool consistency be like? Answer—the consistency of cooked oatmeal, not formed. The passage of large formed stool causes pain. On subsequent bowel movements fear of a painful experience can lead to withholding, which ends up as chronic constipation. Remember, fear is their strongest emotion—it's protective and survival related.

Hopefully at the celebration of his or her first birthday, your toddler does not feed on junk. The association of junk food with this important event, which involves family and community, must not be allowed to happen.

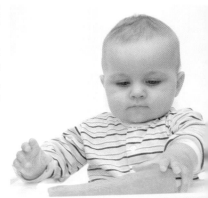

	Food Introduction Schedule	
Eighteen Months	Beans Beets and beet greens Buckwheat Chard Chicken Eggplant Eggs Fish	Garbanzo beans Goat milk yogurt Kelp Other greens (lettuce, mustard, etc.) Rye Tahini
Twenty-one Months	Almond butter Cashew butter Oranges	Pineapple Salmon (wild) Turkey Wheat
Twenty-four to Thirty-six Months	Corn (if no reaction) Cottage cheese Hard cheese Lentils	Peanut butter Sunflower seeds

Caution: Avoid Sugar Overload on the First Birthday

Delay the introduction of refined sugars and other sweets as long as you can. Although it's tempting to put a gigantic cake in front of baby on her first birthday or feed her ice cream when she won't eat anything else, the longer you can put off introducing these foods, the less hooked on them she's likely to become.

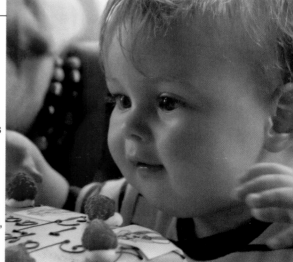

Healthy Eating in the Second Year

ONCE YOUR BABY CAN chew, pick up food between fingers and thumb, and feed himself, your options for feeding dramatically expand. The foods described below are appropriate for children aged fifteen months and beyond or for slightly younger kids with enough teeth to chew foods well.

As a general rule, you can offer your toddler the same foods that are on your plate, made toddler-friendly by cutting them into small pieces. Toddlers love "nibble trays" with a few different choices set apart from one another. Most toddlers do not like their food mixed up, so whenever possible, use plates with compartments for each food. Here are some more tips to keep in mind.

- Use the size of the child's fist as a guideline for portion sizes.

- Steam carrots and other hard veggies and cut them into small chunks.

- Offer soft-cooked beans; try pinto, black, or garbanzo beans—great finger foods! (Soak dried beans overnight, and discard the water they were soaked in before cooking; otherwise, they can produce gas.)

- Grapes are a choking hazard and should be cut into pieces.

- Fruits rich in vitamin C—berries, citrus, melon, and kiwi—are great.

- Nuts aren't a great choice because of the risk of choking. Try nut and seed butters such as almond, cashew, sesame seed (tahini), and macadamia nut butters over peanut butter when possible. Peanuts can harbor aflatoxin, a carcinogenic mold. If you suspect your child has food allergies, delay the introduction of nuts (and any food products containing nuts) until after the age of three.

- Try brown or wild rice cooked with plenty of water so that it's sticky enough to mold into toddler-friendly balls. Roll the balls in a mixture of kelp, garlic powder, and sesame seeds.

- Slow-cooked oatmeal is a healthy breakfast; stir in ground flaxseed (ground in a coffee grinder), a teaspoon of organic maple syrup, fresh or frozen berries, or 1 teaspoon raw honey if your child is over one year of age. (Raw honey from local farms is excellent for pollen allergies.)

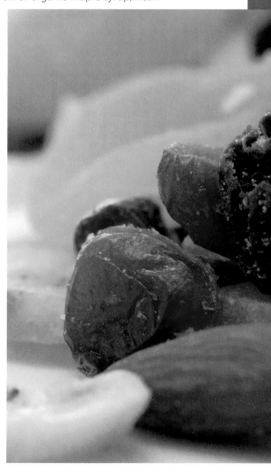

- Dried fruit is a good source of phytonutrients when fresh fruits are out of season. Choose unsulfured dried berries, apricots, and other brightly colored fruits. Stew and puree them for children who aren't ready to chew dried fruit.

- Make your preschooler's noodles whole-grain or rice noodles. Breads and cereals made from whole grains are OK too, but read labels to ensure they aren't loaded with sugar. I prefer sprouted breads such as cinnamon raisin sprouted bread, which is especially good after toasting.

- Keep processed food and junk foods out of the house completely.

- Don't use sweets as a reward or a method for bribing the child into eating more nutritious food. Offer nonfood rewards for good eating habits—a trip to the playground, a game played with mom, or extra hugs and kisses.

HEALTHY HABITS FROM PRESCHOOL TO PRETEEN

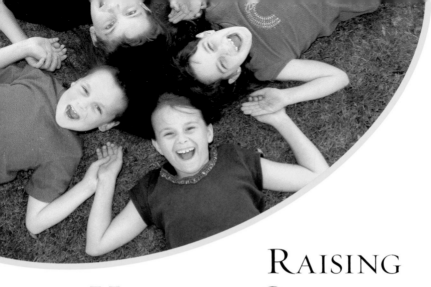

RAISING HEALTHY CHILDREN

WHAT IS A HEALTHY child? Health is a state of complete physical, mental, and social well-being—not merely the absence of disease or infirmity. All modern Western children are at increasing risk of so-called activity-limiting conditions such as asthma, allergies, learning disabilities, ADHD, depression, autism, being overweight, and recurrent bouts of upper respiratory infections. There is a rise in low-birth-weight babies who are at increased risk of long-term illness, disability, and death.

Where once children were at risk from inadequate food, excessive exposure to disease-causing germs, and lack of medicines, many of today's children are born into an overfed, under-germ-exposed, overmedicated, underactive environment. Many are deprived of breast milk as infants and given commercial baby formula that undermines the natural development of their immune system (since approximately two-thirds of the immune system is located in the gastrointestinal tract)—as does the artificially germfree environment in which many children grow up.

Children will naturally clamor for junk foods that are marketed and packaged specifically for them. Don't get in the habit of falling prey to those who profit from marketing directly to children—companies who, in marketing meetings, try to figure out how to optimize "the nag factor" in improving their bottom line. Once your child recognizes that you won't be buying those foods, he'll quit asking for them. Just before the evening meal, when kids are likely to be most hungry, put out a plate of cut-up raw vegetables with healthy low-fat dips such as Galeos dressings or fruit dip.

Getting a child off to a good start in the dietary department will teach him or her good habits for the rest of his or her life. Parents, set the example yourself—you just might make up for your own formula-fed, junk-food, and TV-intensive childhood—to help your child get off on the right foot to a lifetime of good health.

Top Ten "Eat This" Tips for Healthy Kids

Dr. Colbert Approved

1. Don't rush to wean; breast milk is a great addition to baby's diet through the second year of life.

2. Limit processed foods, refined carbohydrates, and fats.

3. Increase fresh, colorful fruits, berries, and vegetables.

4. Use organic foods whenever possible.

5. Purify your household's water.

6. Avoid synthetic chemicals and plastics whenever possible.

7. Judiciously supplement your child's diet with herbs and micronutrients.

8. Make a point of engaging your child in vigorous physical activity every day. (Research shows that overuse of strollers for young children may predispose them to being overweight later on.[1])

9. Get your child out in the sun for fifteen minutes at a time, two to three times a week if possible, or use a supplement that supplies vitamin D.

10. Sit down and eat as a family. Eat on a schedule; children thrive on routine.

A Word From Dr. Cannizzaro: What If My Child Doesn't Like Healthy Foods?

Like babies, kids can be *neophobic*—afraid of new things. "I don't like it" means they haven't tried it enough—it's new. Repeated samplings (even ten or twenty times) might be needed before they'll accept it.

Of course, the ideal situation is that you completely put off introducing refined sugar and other sweets so your child never becomes hooked on them. But if you've already given your kids unhealthy foods, it's never too late to get them on the right eating path. With reform in the home, good choices will be made. It just takes patience as they learn to accept the new healthy foods in their diets. There's more advice on getting your kids to like healthy foods on the next page.

Do You Have a Picky Eater?

If your child is a picky eater, don't worry. This is very common in young children. As long as your child is growing normally and is healthy and energetic, he is probably getting adequate nutrition.

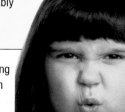

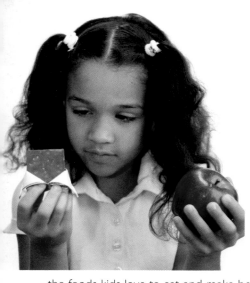

GETTING KIDS TO LOVE FOODS THAT LOVE THEM BACK

CHANGING THE WAY YOU eat is one of the most difficult things for *anyone* to change. Kids are no exception. Parents must review the foods kids love to eat and make better choices of the same food. The transition from junk food to fruits and vegetables might not be easy, but your children's lives may very well depend upon it. Here are five tips to get you started.

1. Involve kids in the decision to eat healthier.

I like a program developed by Dr. David Katz, an epidemiologist at Yale University. It's called "The Nutrition Detectives" and teaches kids to be nutrition detectives and function as spies in the supermarket. The kids use the information they've learned about good nutrition to decide which foods to buy; at home they are allowed to help prepare and even play with their food. All of these things help to engage them in the decisions about their food and to care about what they're eating.

2. Relate healthy eating to activities they love.

Ask your children what they love to do. The answers will probably include things like swimming, basketball, dance, soccer, etc. Ask them next where they get the energy to do these activities—most of them know it's from food. Next, ask them, "Do you want to run fast when you run or jump high when you jump?" Of course they will say that they do. Now you can explain that for a high-performance body, you must feed it high-performance fuel.

3. Relate healthy eating to having fun.

Kids are not experts in chronic disease, but they are experts in fun. They are focused on fun. Teach them the basic message that healthy people have more fun; kids can relate to this. Playing a taste-testing game when their friends are over is a great way to introduce new foods. If a child doesn't like veggies, try steaming them or cutting them up raw and dipping them in their favorite healthy dips, such as hummus. or Galeos dressings.

4. Tell them stories.

You can also teach your kids about healthy eating by telling stories. To reiterate that "you are what you eat," tell them a story about building a wooden house. Ask, "Would you use rotten wood?" The answer, of course, is no. Now relate it to the food they eat, such as sugar and white bread being dead foods like rotten wood.

5. Getting older kids on board.

If you have older children or preteens in your home, try enlisting their help to teach your younger kids how to eat—they won't even realize that they are learning the same eating principles as they teach them to younger siblings or cousins.

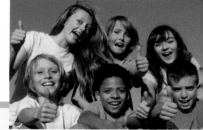

It's important that kids of any age get the message that they don't have to give up the foods they love; we want them to look for foods that love them back, foods that give strength and vitality to grow healthy.

Grocery Store Detectives

Ninety-five percent of our food choices are packaged in bags, boxes, bottles, and cans. Teach your kids the following label-reading tips.

- Don't be fooled by the enticing ads on the front of the package—read the ingredients list on the back. Look for whole grains (good!) and artificial colorings and flavorings (bad!). "Fruit flavors" are not real fruit. Kids don't like to be deceived. Tell them, "You have to look out for you. The makers of these products are not. They simply want you to buy something and will trick you to do it."

- The first ingredient is the most abundant. Some boxed breakfast cereals have as much sugar as a bag of candy. Add the artificial coloring, and, as Dr. Cannizzaro says, "You might as well give your kids jelly beans in milk!" (In fact, these cereals should be labeled cookies or candy, but not cereal.)

- Look for hidden junk in food, such as partially hydrogenated oils, monosodium glutamate (MSG), and high-fructose corn syrup (HFCS). The front of the package may say zero trans fats, but partially hydrogenated oil *is* trans fat. Since the serving size is small, the amount of trans fat meets a criterion of 500 mg or less to allow the manufacturers to say on the front of the package: zero trans fats. If hydrogenated or partially hydrogenated fats are listed in the ingredients list, do not buy the product.

- The longer the ingredient list, generally the worse the food. Choose items with a short list: broccoli (one ingredient).

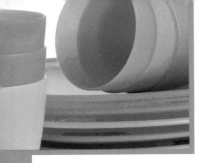

Tips for the Preschool Diet

OFFER PRESCHOOLERS THE SAME foods that are on your plate—made child friendly by cutting the food into smaller pieces. Preschoolers love nibble trays with a few different choices set apart from one another. They don't like their foods mixed up—use plates with compartments for each food. Here are some more tips to keep in mind:

- The meal is the main event. Connecting with your family is the goal. No TV, phone calls, computer, iPod, games, or reading materials at the table.
- Eat fresh, whole, seasonal foods, and involve the kids in the meal plan and preparing the foods.
- Connect your kids to your extended family or cultural background by sharing your family's food traditions. As you cook with your child, share childhood stories of cooking with family members.
- Teach them that balance is the key to living a healthy life and that moderation is the key.
- Train them to notice how they feel after eating too much sugar or other additives.
- Use the time during dinner to learn about each other's day or plan family activities. The point of the meal is to connect with one another. Unpleasant issues or discipline should be saved for later. Always keep the conversation pleasant, and do not reprimand children at meals.
- If eating has become a battle, have your child stay at the dinner table to participate in the family event whether she chooses to eat or not. Avoid power struggles, and instead allow her to enjoy staying emotionally connected with the family.
- Model the eating habits that you hope to instill in your children. Keep in mind the average child sees about ten thousand food commercials per year, with the majority of those for candy, soda, fast food, or sugared cereal. As families, we need to reclaim the art of nutrition.
- Teach your children mindful eating. Pause for a moment and look at the food you're about to put in your mouth. Appreciate it and thank God for providing nourishment for you and your family. Say a brief prayer together before eating and teach your children to express gratitude.

Getting Young Children to Eat Vegetables

If you can grow any vegetables yourself, try to make this part of the time you spend with your kids. Live in an apartment? Try a little herb garden. Sprouting raw nuts, seeds, beans, and legumes, which you can get at your health food store or via mail order, is a wonderful experience for parents to share with children. Simply place the sprouts-to-be in a colander, sprouting bag, or sprouting jar; rinse daily until sprouts shoot out.

Take young children on outings to farms, pick your own produce, pet the cows, and watch the chickens scratch and peck. Show them where their food comes from. Children who see food as a link with nature are more likely to eat natural foods without a fuss.

When Your Kids Want Sweets

Eventually, your child will get a taste of sweets and refined, processed, attractively packaged foods. If it hasn't happened by the time she's in preschool or kindergarten, it will once she gets there. Make it clear that those foods are once-in-a-while foods.

Try creating a schedule where your family has a sweet treat no more than one day a week. "Oh, you want a candy bar? It's not our sweets day—we'll have one on Sunday!" Show your child those days on the calendar; it's also a good way to introduce the days of the week. (But remember you don't want to use sweets or sweets days as a reward! It teaches children to associate sweets with good behavior or with good times, making these comfort foods and therefore making them more enticing.)

Healthy Treat Alternatives

Allow healthful treats like fruit smoothies; a frozen juice pop; home-made granola; plain or organic yogurt with granola, fruit, and a dash of pure maple syrup; frozen or fresh fruit; trail mix; sulfite-free dried fruit; nuts; seeds; or applesauce during snack times any day. If you need something sweet to help get through a car ride or a time when quiet is needed, try sugar-free lollipops made with xylitol. Most health food stores carry them, and they also prevent cavities.

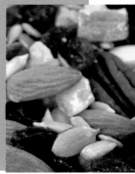

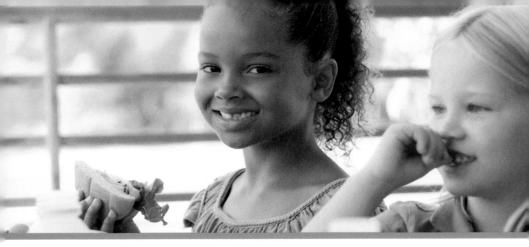

EATING HABITS IN ELEMENTARY SCHOOL

EXPERTS BELIEVE THAT TODAY'S youth are going to be the first generation of Americans to not outlive their parents.[2] Dr. Cannizzaro and I treat increasing numbers of patients who are diabetic and obese in large part due to poor food choices and lack of activity. We are publishing this book as part of a much-needed comprehensive prevention strategy that educates parents like you on how to provide healthy food choices.

Having dinner together in the evening is difficult for today's families. According to a recent Gallop poll, 28 percent of adults with children under the age of eighteen report that they eat dinner together at home seven nights a week—down from 37 percent in 1997. Almost half (47 percent) say their families eat together between four and six times a week, and a quarter (24 percent) say they eat together three or fewer nights a week.[3]

When parents sit down and eat with their children, they are teaching their children, whether they are aware of it or not, and leading by example. They are teaching them what foods to choose, to slow down and enjoy the food, to fellowship, tell stories, and make meals pleasant and something to look forward to. Parents are teaching their children to eat when they are hungry and to stop when they are satisfied and not stuffed. As a parent, you are able to mold and create healthy food habits and choices that actually bring comfort and contentment to your child. This in turn creates good memories that cause lasting impressions on what foods they will choose as they get older.

Teens who eat with their parents consume more fruits and vegetables and drink less soda, according to a recent survey. Additionally, a recent government report revealed that as family dinners declined, teen substance abuse rose. Teens who ate more than five dinners a week with their families were 32 percent less likely to try cigarettes, 45 percent less likely than their peers to try alcohol, and 24 percent less likely to try marijuana.[4]

Ten Benefits of Family Dinners

A report from the National Center on Addiction and Substance Abuse at Columbia University found ten benefits of family dinners. Teens are:

1. Less likely to smoke cigarettes
2. Less likely to drink alcohol
3. Less likely to try marijuana
4. Less likely to have friends who use illicit drugs
5. Less likely to have friends who abuse prescription drugs
6. More likely to get mostly As and Bs at school
7. More likely to say they would confide in one or both parents about a serious problem
8. More likely to report that their parents are proud of them
9. More likely to report lower levels of stress and tension at home
10. More likely to talk to their families during dinner and have the TV off during the meal[5]

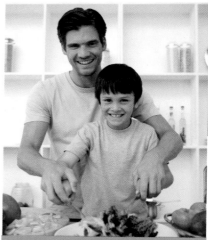

High-Low Conversations

Remember the High-Low Conversation Rule: keep the conversation high at the dinner table. Ask what the best things were that happened to each family member that day. Save the low points of the day for later. Before bedtime is a good time to resolve any problems and offer forgiveness if needed, but don't discuss these problems at the table. Keep mealtimes pleasant and positive.

Breakfast Is Not Optional

A healthy breakfast is the most important meal of the day for your child. A healthy breakfast containing healthy protein, fats, carbohydrates, and fiber will satisfy hunger, provide energy, enable the child to focus, and help prevent obesity. According to research, children who eat breakfast tend to be less overweight than children who don't. A good breakfast is also associated with better concentration, better attention, memory, and achievement in school. A good breakfast is NOT a doughnut, toaster pastry, cereal full of sugar, and a glass of juice.

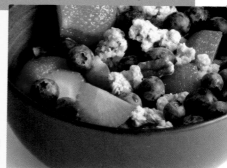

THE SAD STATE OF SCHOOL LUNCHES

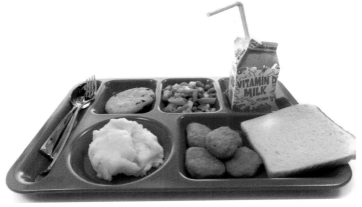

IN OUR LOCAL SCHOOLS a daily choice of pizza, hamburger, french fries, and other low-nutrient foods are offered to our children. Sugar and flour permeate the menu. Beef has eleven ingredients where one would be expected. If your children eat two meals a day at school, like many of today's students, that school lunch program has the ability to influence 66 percent of their meals.

Until these healthier options become a part of school menus, it is up to parents to provide healthy food choices for their school-aged youngsters by providing quick, healthy breakfasts and packing lunches (many kids eat both breakfast and lunch at school these days). Here are some tips to help you provide quick and easy breakfasts and pack healthy school lunches your kids won't want to trade!

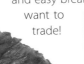

Healthy Snacks

First, remove junk foods, sugary foods, and irresistible foods from your home. Be sure to limit the treats you keep in the house, and put them out of sight or hide them. Keep bowls of fruit, high-fiber crackers (such as Wheat Thins Fiber Select), double-fiber breads or cinnamon raisin sprouted bread, low-fat or nonfat yogurt without fruit syrup, such as vanilla Greek yogurt well stocked in your home. Also, keep baby carrots, celery, and other veggies to be dipped in healthy low-fat dressings such as Galeos dressings from Whole Foods. Nuts, seeds, and nut butters (such as almond butter and natural peanut butter) are excellent choices.

Quick and Healthy Breakfasts

1. High-fiber cereals with low sugar and low-fat or skim milk. Add a handful of nuts (any kind) if your child is not allergic. Also eat one piece of fruit.

2. One to two organic eggs, toasted Ezekiel 4:9 bread with Smart Balance or Just Fruit spreads, one to two slices of nitrite-free turkey bacon, and one piece of fruit.

3. Quaker Oats high-fiber instant oatmeal with berries, nuts and ground flaxseeds added; 8-ounce glass low-fat or skim milk; one piece of fruit.

4. French toast made with cinnamon raisin sprouted bread and pure maple syrup as topping. For each slice of french toast add 1 egg, 1 tsp. vanilla extract, and $1/4$–$1/2$ tsp. cinnamon. Mix ingredients well, coat bread, and cook both sides until golden brown. Also eat one piece of fruit.

5. Whole-wheat buttermilk pancakes with blueberries, blackberries, or raspberries cooked inside them. These are so delicious that children rarely ask for syrup.

6. Toasted sprouted wheat cinnamon raisin bagels with low-fat or nonfat cream cheese; one piece of fruit

7. Breakfast smoothie: mix $1/4$–$1/2$ cup frozen berries of choice; 1 cup nonfat vanilla Greek yogurt or low-fat milk; 2 Tbsp. ground-up flaxseeds, almond butter, or flaxseed oil; $1/2$–1 frozen banana (optional). Add a small amount of low-fat or skim milk if the smoothie is too thick.

Quick, Healthy Lunches

Include a salad or veggie, and a fruit, with each of the lunches below.

1. Black bean soup with brown or wild rice

2. Sandwich made with double-fiber wheat bread or Ezekiel 4:9 bread and turkey, roast beef, or chicken. You may use a small amount of mustard, ketchup, or low-fat mayonnaise. Add lettuce and tomatoes.

3. Stir-fried chicken or beef (prepared the night before) with garlic, curry sauce (or other spice), broccoli, onions, and other veggies. Serve with brown or wild rice. Turn this into a roll-up by wrapping it in an Ezekiel 4:9 tortilla.

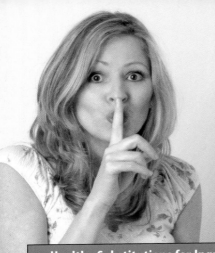

"STEALTH" NUTRITION

UNTIL YOUR KIDS ARE completely on board with healthier eating, you may need to "sneak" some healthier ingredients into their standard favorites. After your kids tell you they love these dishes, you'll have the perfect opportunity to teach them that eating healthily doesn't have to taste bad.

Healthy Substitutions for Ingredients in Foods Your Kids Already Love

Common Ingredient	Healthy Substitution
Bacon	Canadian bacon or turkey bacon (nitrite free)
Bread crumbs	Crushed nuts, rolled oats, or crushed bran cereal
Butter or shortening (for baking)	Canned pumpkin or applesauce for half of the amount called for
Butter or margarine (to prevent sticking)	Olive oil or cooking spray
Butter (for flavor)	Flaxseed oil, almond butter, or other nut butters, Smart Balance
Cheddar or high-fat cheeses	Part-skim mozzarella, provolone, or other low-fat cheese
Milk Chocolate	Dark chocolate
Creamed soups and sauces	Puréed white beans, cauliflower, potatoes, or carrots
Deep-frying, grilling, or microwaving	Stir-frying, baking, toasting, or steaming
Enriched macaroni noodles	Whole-grain or brown rice noodles or pasta
Flour (as a thickening agent)	Arrowroot (This will not be a 1:1 substitution; you will need to play it by ear until you've added enough arrowroot to thicken the sauce to the desired consistency.)
Mayonnaise	Vegenaise or plain low-fat yogurt
Seasoning salt	Herb-only seasonings
Sour cream	Plain low-fat yogurt or cottage cheese with lemon juice or fat-free sour cream
Syrup	Puréed fruit, organic honey, or maple syrup
Vegetable oil (for moisture in baking)	Puréed fruit
Whipped cream (for topping desserts)	Frozen yogurt
Whole or condensed milk	Nonfat milk (skim)
Regular salt	Himalayan sea salt or sea salt

Guilt-Free Spaghetti With Meatballs

Cook whole-wheat spaghetti (not thin spaghetti or angel hair) according to package instructions for al dente, which is typically for about six minutes. (The thinner and more cooked the pasta is, the higher its glycemic index score.) In a bowl, combine 2–6 oz. extra-lean ground beef with an omega-3 egg, chopped onion, roasted minced garlic, Mrs. Dash Italian Blend seasoning mix, granulated garlic, salt, and pepper. Roll into 1-inch meatballs and brown in skillet. Add to Classico or Newman's Own Tomato and Basil Pasta Sauce in saucepan and heat through. Serve over pasta.

Simple Snack Swaps

Regular salad dressings	Low-fat salad dressings; Galeos low-fat salad dressings; ¼ cup extra-virgin olive oil and ¾ cup balsamic vinegar
Fried chicken nuggets	Baked, grilled, or stir-fried chicken breast strips
Regular cheese	Low-fat or part skim milk cheese
Regular yogurt	Low-fat or nonfat Greek yogurt without fruit; choose plain or vanilla and add your own fruit
Potato or tortilla chips	Baked chips
French fries	Oven-baked fries

Sneaking in Healthier Carbs

If your kids are already used to sugary cereals, don't shock their taste buds with a "cold turkey" switch. You'll have more success if you make smaller changes over time. Try mixing whole-grain, unsweetened cereals into their regular cereal and gradually increasing the ratio of healthy to unhealthy cereal over time. Try this same method when making the switch to brown rice, whole-grain flours, and whole-grain pastas. You can also combine mashed white and sweet potatoes for a while to gradually move your family in a healthier direction.

Other "Sneaky" Ways to Add Nutrition to Your Child's Diet

- Add fruit to whole-grain muffins, pancakes, and waffles when you make them.
- Purée veggies like zucchini, carrots, and red or black beans and add them to spaghetti sauce or other tomato-based sauces.
- Substitute plain or Greek yogurt for mayonnaise in most recipes.
- Add spinach (or any green veggies) to blueberry smoothies or other foods with berries. The blueberries will hide both the taste and green coloring of your hidden veggies.
- Add sardines to tuna salad.
- Add grated zucchini to baked goods that call for flaked coconut.
- Add bran to cookies.

WHAT TO DRINK

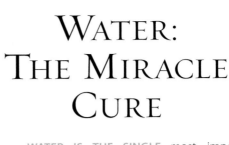

WATER: THE MIRACLE CURE

WATER IS THE SINGLE most important nutrient for our bodies. It is involved in every function of our bodies. You can live five to seven weeks without food, but the average adult can last no more than five days without water.[1]

Many children never drink water. Some don't like the taste of water, or they aren't being taught the importance of drinking it. They live in a mildly dehydrated state with various irritating symptoms and never realize it. I often tell patients that when they have a headache, they don't have a Tylenol deficiency. When they have joint pain, they don't have an Advil deficiency. When they have heartburn, they don't have a Pepcid deficiency, and if they are depressed, they don't have a Prozac deficiency. In each of these cases, their body is often crying out for water.[2]

I treat every patient I see in my practice first with water. Most of my patients get better when they simply drink adequate amounts of water their body is asking for. Drinking sufficient amounts of the right kind of water may also do more to improve your child's health than anything else you can do.

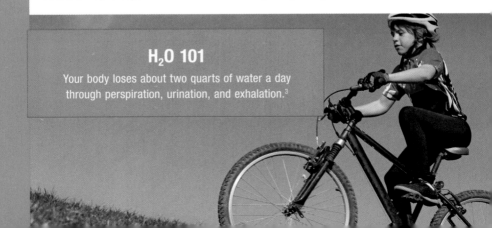

H₂O 101

Your body loses about two quarts of water a day through perspiration, urination, and exhalation.[3]

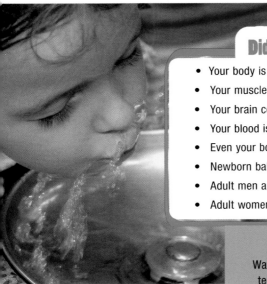

Did You Know...?

- Your body is about 55 to 60 percent water.
- Your muscles are about 75 percent water.
- Your brain cells are about 70 percent water.
- Your blood is approximately 83 percent water.
- Even your bones are approximately 25 percent water.
- Newborn babies are about 78 percent water.
- Adult men are about 60 percent water.
- Adult women are about 55 percent water.[4]

It's a Fact!

Water plays a vital role in regulating body temperature, transporting nutrients and oxygen to cells, removing waste, cushioning joints, and protecting organs and tissues.[5]

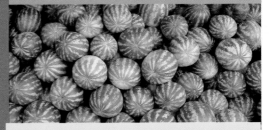

Wet Behind the Ears?

Different people have different percentages of their bodies made up of water. Babies, when they are born, have the highest percentage of water in their bodies, at about 78 percent. What is the water percentage in the body of a one-year-old?

a. 55 percent

b. 62 percent

c. 65 percent

Answer: c. By the age of one year, the percentage of water in the body drops to 65 percent.[6]

Take a Guess

Which food is highest in water content?

a. Watermelon

b. Lettuce

c. Grapefruit

Answer: b. Lettuce. Although all of the foods listed have a high percentage of water content, a half-cup of lettuce has the highest at 95 percent.

WATER: HOW MUCH AND HOW OFTEN?

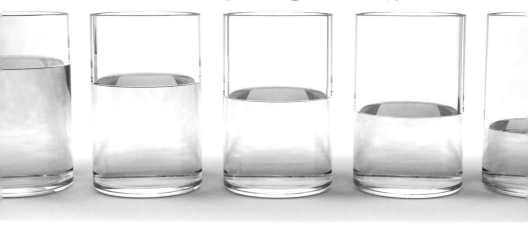

OUR BODIES YEARN FOR pure, clean water. But one of the most common questions I hear is, "How much water should I drink?" I'm going to give you the answer to that question. To determine how much water your body needs, take your body weight (in pounds) and divide it by two. That's how many ounces of water you need every day. The same principle holds true for your child, unless he or she is an infant, in which case you should consult your physician or pediatrician.

For an adult this amounts to two or three quarts a day. Picture a one-gallon container of milk, and imagine it three-quarters full. If you are an average-sized adult, that's about how much water your body needs daily. If you weigh 120 pounds, you will need 60 ounces of water; if 220 pounds, you'll need 110 ounces. For children it will be less, based on their body weight.

But they won't consume it all in liquid form. Simply by eating lots of fruits and vegetables—as they should—they will typically get a quart of water a day. Foods such as bananas are 70 percent water; apples, 80 percent water; tomatoes and watermelons are more than 90 percent water; and lettuce is 95 percent water. Also, milk is predominately water, so infants generally do not require water. Newborns do not need

How Much Should I Drink?

Take your weight in pounds and divide it by two. The result is how many ounces of water you should drink daily.

_____ Weight ÷ 2 = _____ ounces per day

water as breast milk and formula are sufficient. Drinking water is not recommended until around six to twelve months of age. If your child eats an inordinate amount of starches, like breads or pastries, he or she will need more water, because these foods add little water to the body.

When to drink water

Most kids wait until they are thirsty or until they have a dry mouth before they take a drink. By that time they are most likely already mildly dehydrated. A dry mouth is one of the last signs of dehydration.

Other kids only drink during meals—another mistake. When you drink too much with a meal, it washes out the hydrochloric acid, digestive juices, and enzymes in your stomach and intestines, which delays digestion. Fluids, and iced drinks in particular, quench the digestive process similarly to pouring water on a fire.

Your child can drink some water with a meal. I usually drink room-temperature unsweetened tea or bottled water with a slice of lemon or lime squeezed into it. But don't go overboard. Meals are not the time for your child to get most of his or her fluids. Stick to only about 8 ounces with a meal.

Climate Matters

If you live in a warmer or drier climate, your child will need more water. Most of us lose about a pint of water a day through perspiration. Our bodies also lose water through exhalation (about a pint a day) and through urination and stool (about two pints a day).[7] Two pints equal one quart, so our bodies lose about one and a half to two quarts a day. However, this doesn't account for excessive perspiration, especially after vigorous and prolonged exercise. Make sure to weigh your children before and after they participate in sports or activities. For each pound they lose, have them drink about two cups of water.[8]

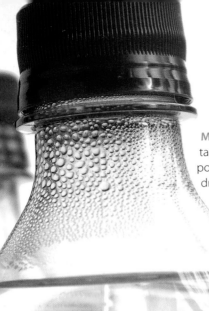

BOTTLED WATER

MANY PEOPLE DRINK BOTTLED water instead of tap water, making bottled water the second most popular beverage in the United States behind soft drinks.[9] People today consume twice as much bottled water as they did a decade ago, and the growth in the bottled water industry is "unparalleled," according to the Beverage Marketing Corporation.[10]

But is bottled water healthier for you and your child? Does that attractive bottle with the pictures of snowy mountains and crystalline streams really mean the water inside is pure?

Less Regulated Than Tap

Bottled water is considered a food; therefore, it is regulated by the FDA. Tap water is regulated by the EPA.[11] The only requirement placed on bottled water is that it be as safe as tap water. But while the EPA makes cities test public drinking water daily, the FDA requires only yearly testing for bottled water.[12] The EPA forbids the presence of bacteria, which indicate the presence of fecal material, but the FDA has no such rule, meaning bottled water can contain fecal bacteria and still be legal.[13]

More Toxins Than Tap

A study of one hundred brands of bottled water showed that a third contained arsenic, trihalomethanes, bacteria, or other contaminants. A fifth contained man-made chemicals, and one contained phthalates at twice the level acceptable in tap water. Two had high levels of fluoride, and two others had coliform bacteria.[14] And if you think that bottled water is lead free, think again. The FDA allows bottled water to contain up to five parts per billion of lead.[15]

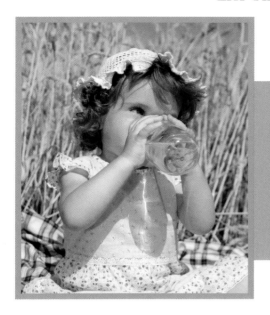

Where Bottled Water Really Comes From

Dasani and Aquafina waters, two of the biggest brands in America, are repro-cessed tap water from cities around the country. One of Aquafina's sources is the Detroit River![16] About one-fourth of bottled water is tap water, according to government and industry estimates.[17]

A Word From Dr. Cannizzaro

I recommend introducing water (1 ounce twice a day) starting at six months. Water purification with catalytic ionization and ultraviolet light processes are ideal.

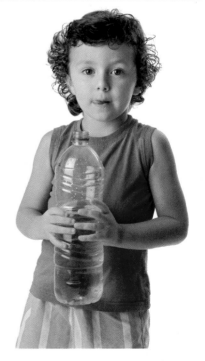

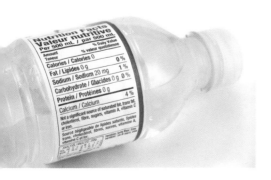

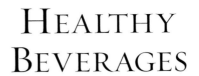

HEALTHY BEVERAGES

UNFORTUNATELY, CHILDREN ARE CHOOSING to drink sodas, juices, smoothies, milk shakes, chocolate milk, or other beverages loaded with sugar. Research has found that when preschool-age children consume sugar-sweetened beverages between meals, this more than doubles their risk of being overweight.[18] Researchers have also found that children ages two to nineteen get up to 15 percent of their total daily calories from beverages that contain sugar.[19] A 12-ounce can of soda typically contains about 8 teaspoons of sugar. Many children are supersizing their sodas and getting about 24 teaspoons of sugar per serving.

Many mothers believe that fruit juice is much healthier than sodas. Well, it is a little healthier because of the vitamin C it contains, but fruit juice usually contains just as much sugar as sodas. Many times the juice is "imitation juice" and contains only about 10 percent real juice. The American Academy of Pediatrics recommends limiting children ages one to six to between 4 and 6 ounces of pure fruit juice a day; children between the ages of seven and eighteen should have a maximum of 8 to 12 ounces a day.[20]

Does Your Child Like Juice?

If your child loves grape, apple, or orange juice, simply dilute the juice with equal parts of water. For example, for 4 ounces of grape juice, add 4 ounces of water. But limit your child's juice intake because juice is high in sugar.

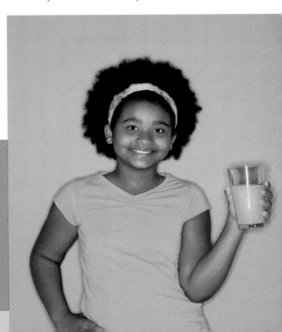

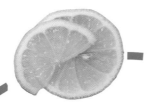

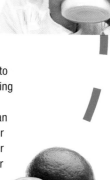

So what beverages are good for children?

Well, we've already discussed water, but milk is also important—unless you are allergic to milk or have excessive mucus or ear infections. One- and two-year-old children need whole milk. School-age children and teens should drink low-fat or skim milk. The 2005 Dietary Guidelines for Americans suggest that children drink at least 16 ounces of milk a day. However, children are drinking significantly less milk than 16 ounces a day and instead are choosing sodas and fruit drinks. I encourage parents to make healthy lemonade, limeade, or ginger ale by squeezing lemons, limes, or ginger and adding stevia to taste. (See Appendix E.) You can also use sparkling water such as San Pellegrino to make lemon, lime, or freshly squeezed ginger drinks, with added stevia, that are similar to 7UP or ginger ale. These are some healthy alternatives to help keep your child at a healthy weight and resistant to disease.

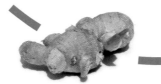

SUPPLEMENTS

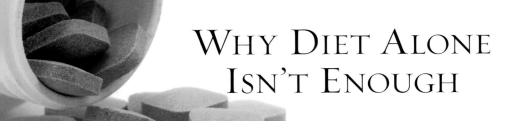

WHY DIET ALONE ISN'T ENOUGH

IN A PERFECT WORLD, the human body would indeed get all the nutrients it needs from food. Ideally, the vitamins and minerals our bodies need to thrive should come through the foods we eat. However, processed foods have been stripped of much of their nutrient content. Cooking and storage are also reasons why our food loses more nutrients. Our toxic environment and toxins in our food, water, and air, as well as our overstressed lifestyles, have increased our nutrient requirements. Even if we were to eat adequate fruits and vegetables, the nutrient content in them has decreased due to our depleted soils.

That's why few, if any, children get the nutrients they need from food alone, even if they eat a completely healthy diet. That's why I recommend supporting a healthy diet with nutritional supplements that can give you the nutrients you are likely missing from your normal diet. Those nutrients are the building blocks of health, and they will protect you against disease. Without these nutritional supplements, you are likely to have nutrient deficiencies.

It's extremely difficult to provide all the nutrition your child's body needs from diet alone. As I mentioned above, today's soil has fewer nutrients in it than ever before. When soil has fewer nutrients, so do the things that grow in it. According to the 1992 Earth Summit, North America has the worst soil in the world—85 percent of vital minerals have been depleted from it.[1] People noticed this trend as far back as 1936, when the U.S. Senate issued Document 246, which said that impoverished soil in the United States no longer provided plant foods with minerals needed for human nourishment.[2] These losses in soil nutrients eventually will have a significant impact on your child's health.

To be healthy, your child almost certainly needs to start taking nutritional supplements. Which ones to take, in what quantities, and at what age will be the subject of the rest of this chapter.

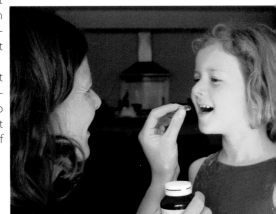

Enzymes and Your Child's Digestion

Poor digestion is another reason people often need nutritional supplements. It's not merely what your child *eats* but what he *assimilates* and *absorbs* into his body that counts. One reason for poor digestion is a lack of enzymes in the diet. Enzymes are essential to the digestion, assimilation, and absorption of food, and there are several steps you can take to help ensure your child has enough enzymes for normal digestion:

1. Avoid highly processed food that is void of enzymes.
2. Consume more raw or slightly steamed vegetables and fruits that are loaded with enzymes.
3. Make sure he chews his food properly, allowing salivary enzymes to help break down the food.
4. Don't cook his food at high temperatures, which destroys the enzymes in the food.
5. Don't allow him to consume excessive amounts of fluids with his meals, which washes out his enzymes.

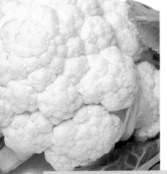

Where Have All the Nutrients Gone?

Comparing the USDA handbook of 1972 to the USDA food tables of today reveals dramatic reductions in nutrient content. Nearly half of the calcium and vitamin A in broccoli have disappeared. The vitamin A content in collard greens has fallen to nearly half its previous levels; potassium dropped from 400 mg to 170 mg, and magnesium fell from 57 mg to only 9 mg. Cauliflower lost almost half of its vitamin C along with its thiamine and riboflavin. The calcium in pineapple went from 17 mg to 7 mg.[3]

A Word From Dr. Cannizzaro: Why Whole Foods Are Best

A whole food does not contain a huge amount of any one nutrient—rather whole foods contain small amounts of numerous nutrients that work together in synergistic balance. By eating whole foods, your child brings this synergy into her body. No man-made multi-nutrient formula can contain all of the vital compounds your child needs to consume, because metabolically necessary nutrients are yet to be discovered and because it is impossible to re-create nature's synergy in a laboratory. However, since it's difficult to consume enough (five to twelve servings) fruit and vegetables on a daily basis, a concentrated whole-food micronutrient supplement is an important addition to a balanced, healthy diet. (See Appendix E.)

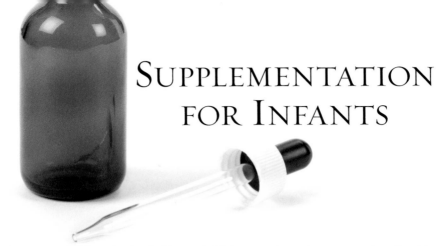

SUPPLEMENTATION FOR INFANTS

I AM OFTEN ASKED whether babies and children need supplements, such as fluoride and other nutrients. On pages 49–50 I provide a list of supplements you can add to commercial baby formulas to make them healthier. Here are my recommendations for additional supplements for both breast-fed and formula-fed babies.

Iron plays a key role in human life as a component of a number of proteins, including hemoglobin, which is critical for the transport of oxygen and electrons to tissues throughout the body. Iron deficiency is the most common single-nutrient deficiency in infants.

Breast-fed babies (who are fed breast milk exclusively through the first six months of life) are considered to have adequate iron intake. Although the iron content of human milk is low, it has been shown to be highly bioavailable (easily absorbed and assimilated by the baby's body). Babies use more than 50 percent of the iron in breast milk but less than 12 percent of that in infant formula due to lower bioavailability. The iron in iron-fortified baby cereals is also of low bioavailability. Therefore, I usually make the following recommendations:

- Formula-fed infants should be provided only iron-fortified formulas, and only iron-fortified formulas should be used for weaning or supplementing breast milk for all infants younger than twelve months.

- Iron supplements are recommended before six months of age for breast-fed infants born with low iron stores due to preterm birth and/ or low birth weight.

- Breast-fed infants need a supplemental source of iron starting at around six months of age, preferably from complementary foods. Iron-fortified infant cereal and/or meats are recommended as good sources for this purpose. If a full-term, breast-fed infant is unable to consume sufficient iron from dietary sources after six months of age, supplemental iron should be used.

Vitamin D's major function is to help the body absorb adequate calcium and phosphorus from the diet. We obtain vitamin D in two ways:

1. Endogenously: our bodies produce vitamin D_3 from exposure to sunlight.

2. Exogenously: we receive vitamin D_3 from dietary sources such as fortified milk and other fortified food products and fish.

Breast-fed infants obtain most of their vitamin D from the breast milk, but mom's exposure to sunlight is usually limited and the vitamin D level in human milk is usually low.

Infant formula is fortified with 400 IU of vitamin D_3; however, vitamin D levels in infants who drink fortified formula are frequently below acceptable levels.

Vitamin D_3 deficiency in infants and children results in inadequate mineralization of the skeleton. This can ultimately cause rickets, which presents with a variety of bone deformations.

For these reasons, the American Academy of Pediatrics Committee on Nutrition recommends that all breast-fed infants receive a dietary supplement of 400 IU a day of vitamin D. I recommend vitamin D_3 supplements for all of my patients beginning at birth with 400 IU per day. (See Appendix E.) Adjustments in dosage are made based on measured vitamin D_3 levels in the bloodstream (50–100 ng/ml is the optimal range).

A Word From Dr. Cannizzaro: What If Your Water Isn't Fluoridated?

Fluoride is considered a nonessential nutrient. Its incorporation into teeth during their development can help prevent dental cavities later in life. I do not recommend supplementation of fluoride at all. While fluoride does help to prevent tooth decay, especially in children, it also partially inhibits approximately a hundred different enzymes in the body. I advise parents to provide foods rich in fluorine into the diet when solid foods are begun. All of these foods must be consumed raw. At an appropriate age after six months the following foods can be included in smoothies: raw saltwater fish, seaweed, goat's milk, sprouted rye seeds, avocado, parsley, and black-eyed peas.

SUPPLEMENTATION DURING CHILDHOOD

WHEN PARENTS QUESTION THE need for supplements among preschool and school-aged children, I often tell them to first watch their child's intake of foods over a few months. If they resist eating certain foods on a regular basis, a supplement of the specific vitamins provided by those foods may be in order. Talk to your pediatrician about supplementing to meet your child's individual needs.

I recommend that most children take a quality multivitamin or whole-food multivitamin that includes the key nutrients listed on these pages, vitamin D_3, a pharmaceutical-grade fish oil supplement, and occasionally a good probiotic (see pages 95–96) to support a balanced diet and contribute to your child's health. I usually start these supplements between one and two years of age. Check with your pediatrician for his or her recommendations.

Calcium

Childhood is a time of critical growth and development, with adequate calcium intake being essential for bone mass development. In girls, peak calcium absorption and deposition in bones occur at or near menarche. At that time, the bone calcium deposition rate is approximately five times that of adulthood, and calcium intake of less than 1,000 mg a day is associated with lower bone mineral density. The decline in bone calcium deposition rate is gradual after menarche. The chart on this page presents the average calcium intakes and Adequate Intake (AI) levels for children. The data indicate that, on average, only children under eight years of age are meeting their recommended calcium intake. Although it is best to get as much calcium as possible from foods because these foods also provide other nutrients that aid your child's body in using calcium, supplementation may be appropriate for children who do not eat sufficient amounts of calcium-rich foods.

Mean Calcium Intakes and Recommended Adequate Intake (AI) Levels for U.S. Children						
	1–3 yrs	**4–8 yrs**	**9–13 yrs**		**14–18 yrs**	
			Girls	**Boys**	**Girls**	**Boys**
Mean Intake	793 mg/d	838 mg/d	918 mg/d	1025 mg/d	753 mg/d	1169 mg/d
AI	500 mg/d	800 mg/d	1300 mg/d	1300 mg/d	1300 mg/d	1300 mg/d

Vitamin D_3

According to researchers at Albert Einstein College of Medicine, seven out of ten U.S. children have low levels of vitamin D_3, raising the risk of bone and heart disease. Vitamin D is critically important for growth and for the normal development of bones and teeth. It may protect against prostate and breast cancer. The higher the vitamin D levels in the blood, the lower the risk for colon and colorectal cancers.[4]

Remember, sun exposure is the most important source of vitamin D, because the skin synthesizes vitamin D in response to UV rays. The widespread use of sunscreen has worsened the epidemic of low vitamin D_3 in our children. I recommend that parents allow their children to have ten to fifteen minutes in the sun before applying sunscreen (unless they burn easily) so that their bodies will be able to make vitamin D.

There are very few good dietary sources of vitamin D. Cod liver oil offers a whopping 1,360 IU per tablespoon. However, I believe a better choice for your child is a high-quality, pharmaceutical-grade fish oil and a supplement of vitamin D_3. The American Academy of Pediatrics recommends that infants, children, and teens should take 400 IU a day of vitamin D in supplement form.

Omega-3 fats

Pharmaceutical-grade fish oil is extremely important for infants, children, and teens. Realize that many deadly degenerative diseases are inflammatory, and fish oil is able to decrease inflammation significantly. By decreasing inflammation, fish oil is able to help treat and prevent conditions such as cancer, heart disease, rheumatoid arthritis, psoriasis, migraine headaches, allergies, Alzheimer's disease, and even diabetes. Fish oil also helps to balance and stabilize neurotransmitters in the brain, which may be helpful in patients with attention deficit disorder, depression, and bipolar disorder.

Multivitamin

Choose a comprehensive multivitamin that has at least 100 percent of the daily reference intake (DRI) of vitamin A, vitamin B_1 (thiamine), vitamin B_2 (riboflavin), vitamin B_3 (niacin), vitamin B_5 (pantothenic acid), vitamin B_6 (pyridoxine), vitamin B_{12}, biotin, folic acid, vitamin C, vitamin D, vitamin E, and vitamin K. Minerals should also be included in your child's multivitamin: boron, calcium, chromium, cobalt, copper, iodine, iron, magnesium, manganese, molybdenum, phosphorous, potassium, selenium, silicon, sodium, sulfur, vanadium, and zinc.

Chewable vitamins, capsules, and powders are available if your child has trouble swallowing the tablet form. To avoid upset stomach, start slowly, giving your child half of the recommended amount after meals. Increase the amount according your child's tolerance, but don't exceed 100 percent of the DRI. (See Appendix D for DRI of vitamins and minerals for children at various ages.) I usually recommend starting a quality multivitamin between the ages of one and two, or as recommended by your pediatrician.

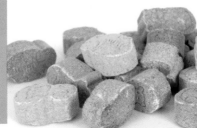

Probiotics: Why Friendly Bacteria Are Essential to Your Child's Health

PROBIOTICS ARE ESPECIALLY IMPORTANT if your child has been on antibiotics (for ear infections, sinus infections, etc.). One of the common side effects of treatment with antibiotics (especially the broad-spectrum type) is that both good and bad bacteria are killed off, opening the door to bacterial and yeast overgrowth and gastrointestinal distress, particularly diarrhea. But probiotics can help restore bacterial balance and prevent other antibiotic-associated side affects.

In one double-blind study, 98 patients taking the antibiotic ampicillin were divided into two groups, one receiving a Lactobacilli supplement while the other group received a placebo. There were no cases of ampicillin-induced diarrhea in the group receiving Lactobacilli, while 14 percent of the placebo group had diarrhea as a result of the antibiotics. Another study involved 27 patients with ear, sinus, or throat infections who were given the antibiotic amoxicillin/clavulanate; some of the patients were also given L. acidophilus. According to the researchers, there was "a significant decrease in patient complaints of gastrointestinal side effects and yeast superinfection" in the group given L. acidophilus supplements.[5]

Using probiotic supplements

Here are some pointers when using probiotics:

- Start low, go slow. Infants can start with 4 or 5 billion CFUs per day and increase gradually to whatever level helps them have better stools and sleep, and less colic, diaper rash, and spit-ups. Children can start at 8 billion CFUs and gradually increase to a level that improves their bowel habits. Some children need 20–40 billion CFUs daily during therapeutic dosing.

- Babies need Bifido strains (like Bifido infantis, Bifado bifidum, Bifido breve) and Lactobacillus acidophilus, which are among the first organisms that typically colonize the human gut. After age two or three, different strains of Lactobacillus (thermophilus, casei, rhamnosus, and others) may become more important while Bifido strains become less so.

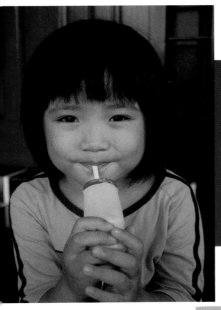

Probiotic Yogurt Drinks Reduce Rate of Illness in Daycares

In 2010, Georgetown University School of Medicine researchers who studied a popular probiotic yogurt-like drink found that it reduced the rate of ear infections, sinusitis, flu and diarrhea in daycare children by 19 percent. The study, titled DRINK (Decreasing the Rates of Illness in Kids), was a randomized, double-blind, placebo-controlled study of 638 healthy children aged three to six who attended school five days a week.[6]

A Word from Dr. Cannizzaro: Go Probiotic From Birth

A study of 154 newborns found that L. acidophilus given shortly after birth encouraged the growth of normal intestinal flora and reduced the number of infections and inflammatory diseases in those infants. Another study demonstrated the L. acidophilus prevents the attachment of harmful bacteria to human intestinal cells, thus providing a barrier against these bacteria in the digestive system.[7] In my practice, I have parents begin supplementing probiotics at birth.

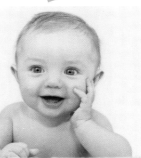

EXERCISE

BENEFITS OF REGULAR PHYSICAL ACTIVITY

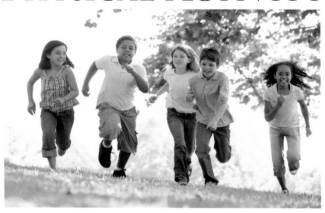

MANY CHILDREN ARE SPENDING less time being active and more time playing video games, being on computers, watching TV, and going to movies. As a result, they are gaining weight and increasing their risk of many adult diseases, including high blood pressure, type 2 diabetes, high cholesterol, fatty liver, heart disease, sleep apnea, acid reflux, and cancer.

The very word *exercise* stresses out many children. Those children who are overweight and/or obese are more prone to feel embarrassed and anxious and to dread exercise. They may have been picked on by other kids or taunted by a coach or PE instructor. Children instead need to view activity as fun. Playing at the playground, swinging on the swing or monkey bars, skating, riding bikes, hiking, playing Wii sports, dancing, swimming, and especially doing these activities as a family are very enjoyable, creating wonderful memories and strengthening family bonds.

On the next few pages I'll tell you about more benefits of regular physical activity.

1. Activity prevents cancer.

Studies show that approximately one-third of cancer deaths can be linked to diet and sedentary lifestyles.[1] Simple movement and exercise decrease the risk of certain cancers such as breast, colon, and possibly endometrial and prostate cancers.[2] In 2005, the National Cancer Institute reported that "physical activity at work or during leisure time is linked to a 50 percent lower risk of getting colon cancer."[3] A study published in the *Journal of the American Medical Association* found that women who engaged in the equivalent of brisk walking for about one to two hours per week decreased their risk of breast cancer by 18 percent compared with inactive women.[4]

2. Activity prevents heart attacks and heart disease.

Cardiovascular disease is the most common cause of death in the United States today.[5] Exercise protects you against it. All kinds of studies show that moderate regular exercise is perhaps one of the most important deterrents of heart-related problems. It also decreases the risk of developing hypertension.

3. Activity improves lymphatic flow.

The lymphatic system is a major microbe crime fighter and cellular garbage collector in the body. It removes toxins and cellular waste, and it "keeps the peace" by rounding up bacteria, viruses, and other bad guys, bringing them to the lymph nodes, where they are killed by white blood cells. Lymphatic fluid is so important that your body contains about three times more lymph than blood. The lymphatic fluid moves around via very small vessels, which usually run alongside small veins and arteries and nerves.

But the lymphatic system has a challenge: it is circulated by muscle contractions, not by your heartbeat. When you don't move, the lymphatic system becomes sluggish. But aerobic exercise can triple the rate of lymphatic flow. That means that the lymphatic system—your in-house police force and cellular garbage collector—does a much better job protecting your body from attack and removing cellular trash.

> ## Activity and Health Fitness
>
> Regular activity improves cardiovascular fitness, improves immune function, helps to lower blood pressure and cholesterol levels, builds strong bones, improves lung function, increases muscle strength and endurance, and enables you and your child to maintain a healthy weight.

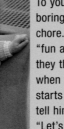

Let's Have Fun!

To your child, the very word *exercise* may sound boring, difficult, and not fun—like a dreaded chore. For that reason I teach parents to call it a "fun activity." Children are very motivated when they think something is fun and involves play. So when your child comes home from school and starts to play video games, resist the urge to tell him to go outside and exercise. Instead say, "Let's go outside and play." Lead by example.

BENEFITS OF REGULAR PHYSICAL ACTIVITY (CONTINUED)

4. Activity helps your child cope with stress.

Regular activity enhances neurotransmitter production and helps to lower cortisol levels, which helps your child feel less stressed. One researcher conducted an experiment with laboratory rats. He took some rats, shocked them with electrodes, shone bright lights, and played loud noises to them around the clock. At the end of one month, all the rats were dead from the stress. He then took another group of rats and made them exercise on a treadmill. After they were well exercised, he subjected them to a month of the same shocks, noises, and lights. These rats didn't die—they ran around well and healthy.[6] If life is stressing your child out, it's time to add activity to your day. Activity helps to burn off those stress chemicals.

5. Activity promotes weight loss and decreases appetite.

Aerobic activity such as brisk walking and cycling is an effective way to lose weight and keep it off. The word *aerobic* means "in the presence of air or oxygen." Aerobic activity is simply movement that strengthens the lungs and the heart. It involves steady, continuous movements that work large muscle groups in repetitive motion for at least twenty minutes. The key point for weight loss with aerobic activity is to maintain a moderate pace that triggers your body to burn fat as its preferred fuel.

Moderate aerobic activity is also quite effective at decreasing your appetite. Daily activity improves your ability to cope with stress by lowering the stress hormone cortisol; therefore, you are usually less likely to be a stress eater. Regular activity also raises serotonin levels, which helps to reduce cravings for sweets and carbohydrates.

6. Activity may help prevent type 2 diabetes and help control blood sugar in diabetics.

Activity holds special benefits for diabetics. By helping muscles to take up glucose from the bloodstream and use it for energy, activity prevents sugar from accumulating in the blood. By burning calories, activity helps control weight, which is also an important factor in the management of type 2 diabetes. Activity is also very important for individuals with type 1 diabetes; it helps to lower insulin requirements and improves the body's ability to use insulin. Multiple studies have shown that those who have a physically active lifestyle are less prone to develop type 2 diabetes.

7. Activity increases perspiration.

Many children would rather be in an air-conditioned home playing a video game or watching TV. God actually told Adam that he would work by the sweat of his brow. Sweating is one of the body's ways of getting rid of waste products. The skin has been called "the third kidney" because it releases so many toxins from the body. It is able to release toxins, including pesticides, solvents, heavy metals, urea, and lactic acid from the body. Activity and perspiration improve circulation to the skin and help remove cellular waste. At normal activity levels, people lose two to three cups of water a day in perspiration. But during an hour of vigorous activity, people sweat out approximately a quart of water.[7]

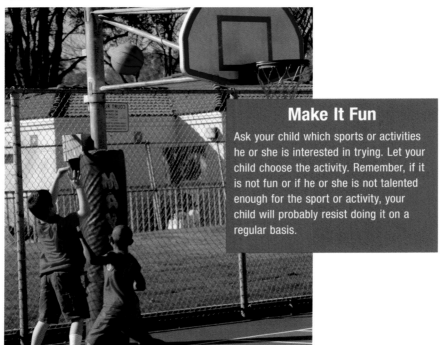

Make It Fun

Ask your child which sports or activities he or she is interested in trying. Let your child choose the activity. Remember, if it is not fun or if he or she is not talented enough for the sport or activity, your child will probably resist doing it on a regular basis.

BENEFITS OF REGULAR PHYSICAL ACTIVITY (CONTINUED)

8. Activity builds strong bones.

Bone density screening has gone high-tech, and as a result, more and more researchers can now measure the effects of various factors in the bone-building process and prevention of osteoporosis. Their research shows that exercise works better than calcium in building strong bones. "Although calcium intake is often cited as the most important factor for healthy bones, our study suggests that exercise is really the predominant lifestyle determinant of bone strength in young women," said Tom Lloyd, PhD, an epidemiologist with the Penn State University College of Medicine, whose findings were reported in the *Journal of Pediatrics*.[8] Exercise slows mineral loss from bones and helps provide strength to your bones and muscles. Weight-bearing exercises actually stimulate the growth of new bone.

9. Activity improves your digestion and promotes regular bowel movements.

Activity helps prevent constipation.[9] Studies have shown that physical activity may help to ease digestion problems and problems with the GI tract. That's the conclusion of a study in an October 2005 issue of *Clinical Gastroenterology and Hepatology*. The study of 1,801 men and women found that obese people who got some form of physical activity were less likely to suffer GI problems than inactive obese people. "It is well documented that maintaining a healthy diet and regular physical activity can benefit GI health," study author Rona L. Levy, a professor at the University of Washington in Seattle, said.[10]

Playing Together

If your children's friends are active and participate in sports, your child will also be more likely to be active and participate in sports.

10. Activity gives you restful sleep.

One of the best ways to improve the quality of your sleep is to be active during the day. Researchers found that women who participated in forty-five minutes of aerobics in the morning were about 70 percent less likely to have trouble sleeping than those who exercised less.[11] You shouldn't exercise within three hours of bedtime because it can cause insomnia; however, stretching and relaxing your muscles at any time of the day have also been shown to make people 30 percent less likely to have trouble sleeping.[12]

11. Activity helps prevent colds and flu.

Research shows that aerobic exercise such as brisk walking, jogging, or cycling boosts the body's defenses against viruses and bacteria during the cold and flu season. Too much exercise can increase your risk of infection, but moderate amounts (thirty minutes, three to four times per week) produce positive results by increasing the circulation of immune cells from bone marrow, the lungs, and the spleen.[13]

12. Activity reduces depression.

Although it is rare, depression can affect kids as young as three years old. If your child is depressed, getting involved in regular physical activity can be a part of the solution; it has been shown to boost the mood in study after study. Regular activity increases serotonin and dopamine levels, which helps to relieve symptoms of anxiety and depression.

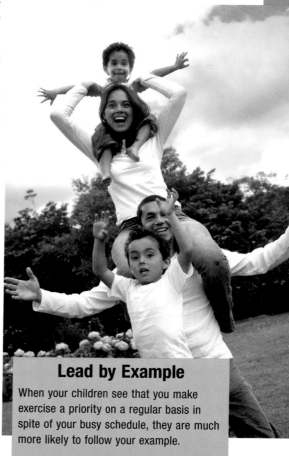

Lead by Example

When your children see that you make exercise a priority on a regular basis in spite of your busy schedule, they are much more likely to follow your example.

Benefits of Regular Physical Activity (continued)

13. Activity increases lung capacity.

As we age, our lung capacity diminishes. Cardiovascular activity and exercise can combat this because activity exercise increases lung capacity. So while our lung capacity may continue to diminish, it does so at a slower pace.[14]

14. Activity alleviates pain.

It might sound crazy to suggest exercising when you are in pain, but regular exercise is a bigger pain-fighting weapon than you might think. Aerobic exercise causes the release of endorphins, which are morphinelike molecules produced by the body. In an article published by the Mayo Clinic, it was reported that regular exercise actually reduces chronic pain for many people. The article quotes Dr. Edward Laskowski of Mayo Clinic as saying, "Years ago, people who were in pain were told to rest, but now we know the exact opposite is true. When you rest, you become deconditioned—which may actually contribute to chronic pain."[15]

15. Activity increases your energy level.

Aerobic activity in your target heart rate range will actually increase your energy. Most people have the excuse that they are simply too tired to exercise; they don't realize that regular aerobic exercise can dramatically increase their energy.[16]

Let's Recap: The Perks of Regular Activity

In case you needed a reminder, here are just a few of the tremendous benefits that come with regular exercise:

- It decreases the risk of heart disease and stroke, as well as the development of hypertension.
- It helps prevent type 2 diabetes.
- It helps protect you from developing certain types of cancer.
- It helps prevent osteoporosis and aids in maintaining healthy bones.
- It helps prevent arthritis and aids in maintaining healthy joints.
- It increases perspiration.
- It improves your mood and reduces the symptoms of anxiety and depression.
- It increases energy and mental alertness.
- It improves your digestion and promotes regular bowel movements.
- It gives you restful sleep.
- It helps prevent colds and flu.
- It alleviates pain.
- It increases lung capacity.
- It helps you cope with stress.
- It improves lymphatic flow.

And the health benefit you likely already knew about...

- It promotes weight loss and decreases appetite!

Family Fun

Choose fun activities to do with your child, such as Wii sports, the game Twister, mini trampoline, Hula hoops, indoor playgrounds at fast-food restaurants (just choose healthy meals), biking, roller blading, swimming, and hiking—and have fun!

Did You Know...?

Researchers at the University of California in San Francisco studied 2,379 girls and found that those whose parents exercised three or more times a week were 50 percent more active than girls whose parents were inactive. And they remained more active than the other girls for nine years.[17]

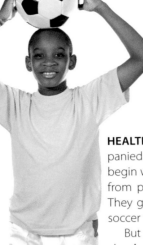

HEALTHY KIDS ARE PHYSICALLY FIT KIDS

HEALTHY EATING IS NOT enough to conquer obesity; it must be accompanied by an active lifestyle. I'm not suggesting you have your child begin working out on a treadmill or lifting weights. Kids can get exercise from playing and being physically active (riding bikes or playing tag). They get added exercise when they take PE classes at school or join a soccer team or dance class.

But you can't assume your child is automatically getting enough exercise. According to the Kaiser Family Foundation, children watch about three hours of television a day, and the average kid spends more than five hours focusing on all media combined (TV, videos, DVDs, computers, and video games). The American Academy of Pediatrics (AAP) recommends that children under the age of 2 years watch no TV at all and that screen time should be limited to no more than 1–2 hours of *quality programming* a day for kids 2 years and older. The AAP suggest that infants and young children should not be inactive for prolonged periods of time (no more than 1 hour during their awake hours), and school-age children should not be inactive for more than 2 hours at a time.

Again, you lead the way with your example. So if you notice your child spending inordinate amounts of time on the couch or playing video games, don't just tell him to go ride his bike while you reach for the remote control—ride bikes with him! Other activities kids and parents can do together include walking the dog; playing catch, volleyball, kickball, or badminton in the backyard; taking a picnic lunch to the park; and joining the YMCA or a health club with family-style fitness programs. (For more information on exercise, please refer to my book *Get Fit and Live!*)

Benefits of Rebounding

Albert E. Carter, author of *Rebound Exercise: The Ultimate Exercise for the New Millennium*, has experienced firsthand the various health benefits of rebounding throughout his life. He can perform 100 hundred push-ups and has never lifted weights in his life. He taught both of his children to rebound from a very early age. His son, Daren, was able to do 429 sit-ups the first time he was challenged (in the first grade), and his daughter, Wendy, was able to do 476 sit-ups without stopping. She beat all the boys in her sixth grade class in arm wrestling even though she had never arm wrestled before! It's interesting that the only exercise they did was to jump on a trampoline.

In addition to strengthening your muscles, rebounding is becoming more recognized for its benefits in fighting cancer due to the way it helps improve your body's lymphatic flow. So get a mini or large trampoline and have fun!

The Three Elements of Fitness

1. **Aerobic exercise:** Your child develops endurance when he regularly engages in aerobic activity.

2. **Anaerobic exercise:** Anaerobics are strengthening and toning exercises. Your child doesn't need to start a weight-training program to develop strength. He simply needs to be playing instead of watching TV. The climbing, running, jumping, wrestling, tumbling, and handstands that children naturally incorporate into their playtime will adequately strengthen their growing muscles. However, you can make a fun obstacle course using push-ups, sit-ups, pull-ups, and other exercises if you feel your child needs additional toning and strengthening. Or take your child to the playground to play on the monkey bars. It's fun and builds strength.

3. **Flexibility and posture exercises:** Stretching is the best way to develop flexibility because it allows your child's muscles and joints to extend to their full range of motion. To get your kids to stretch, have them stand on tiptoe and reach for the sky, bend over and touch their toes while keeping their legs straight, do a split, or do a cartwheel.

Certain Video Games *Can* Burn Calories

WebMD.com recently reported that a third of the Wii sports video and fitness games burn as many calories as moderate-intensity exercises like brisk walking. I believe that getting out and involving your child in real physical activity is still the best way to get fit, but this research shows that any form of activity, even the video variety, is better than none. Consider having a family fun night playing sports together on your Wii instead of letting your children sit and play video games all evening.

How Much Is Enough?

The National Association for Sport and Physical Education (NASPE) offers these activity guidelines for infants, toddlers, preschoolers, and school-age kids:

Age	Minimum Daily Activity	Comments
Infant	No specific requirements	Physical activity should encourage motor development
Toddler	1½ hours	30 minutes planned physical activity **AND** 60 minutes unstructured physical activity (free play)
Preschooler	2 hours	60 minutes planned physical activity **AND** 60 minutes unstructured physical activity (free play)
School age	1 hour or more	Break up into bouts of 15 minutes or more

CREATING A HEALTHY HOME

Toxins in Food

ALMOST ALL NON-ORGANICALLY GROWN produce may be tainted by pesticides, herbicides, parasites, and chemicals. These toxins and microbes find their way into our food supply—and into our bodies. If we don't feed our kids organic foods, the metabolites of toxins are usually found in their bloodstream.

Fatty animal products such as processed meats and fatty meats should be limited or eliminated from a child's diet; choose more organic lean meats. If organic meat is too expensive, then always choose the leanest cuts of meat and the breast of chicken and turkey, making sure to remove the skin. Animals concentrate chemicals and toxins mainly in their fatty tissues from eating the grain and grasses contaminated with chemicals (such as pesticides and herbicides). Organically grown plants build a natural defense system against chemicals and pests to survive, and we benefit all the more by eating these plants. Kids simply must eat more organic.

Although much of our food and water supply may contain toxins, we can detoxify our bodies by switching to an alkalinizing diet rich in fresh organic fruits and vegetables. Alkalinizing foods help to raise the pH of the tissues, enabling the body to release more toxins, whereas acidic foods cause the body to slow this process.

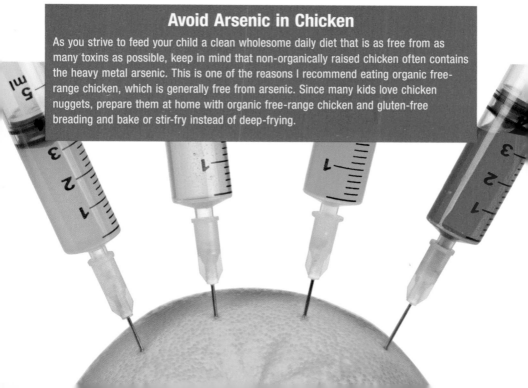

Avoid Arsenic in Chicken

As you strive to feed your child a clean wholesome daily diet that is as free from as many toxins as possible, keep in mind that non-organically raised chicken often contains the heavy metal arsenic. This is one of the reasons I recommend eating organic free-range chicken, which is generally free from arsenic. Since many kids love chicken nuggets, prepare them at home with organic free-range chicken and gluten-free breading and bake or stir-fry instead of deep-frying.

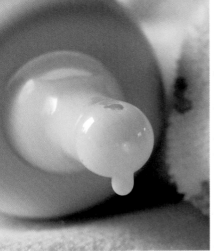

Toxins in breast milk

Chemicals are typically used in food, prescription drugs, some supplements, household products, personal products, and lawn care products. That's why high levels of toxic contaminants have been found in three unlikely places: umbilical cord blood, newborn babies, and breast milk. Contaminants include rocket fuel, flame retardant, dry cleaning fluid.

Nineteen percent of women in their child-bearing years have blood levels of mercury (a neurotoxin) over 5.8, with 5 being the threshold for harmful health effects.[1] If you're thinking about conceiving, you might want to find a doctor who offers a preconception detox program, which helps the body unburden itself of toxic substances through changes in diet, use of herbs (such as cilantro) and other supplements, chelation therapy, zeolites, infrared saunas, glutathione-boosting supplements, and so forth.

Once you are pregnant, these methods must not be used. You must keep the flow of nutrients at optimal levels while empowering the natural pathways of detoxification and digestion to move toxins out of the body through routes other than breast milk. Also, do not get your amalgam fillings (silver fillings) either removed or replaced during pregnancy since they are high in mercury.

Note

If you are reading this while breast-feeding your child without undergoing any type of detox treatment, do not wonder if you should stop breast-feeding. Rest assured that the benefits of your breast milk are helping your child far more than the chemicals in it are hurting.

Quick Quiz

Tainted Breast Milk

When compared to nursing mothers who don't eat meat, how much more pesticide contamination do nursing mothers who eat meat have in their breast milk?

- a. Twice as much

- b. Thirty-five times as much

- c. Ten times as much

(Just another reason to choose organic.)
Answer: b. Thirty-five times as much.[2]

How to Reduce Toxins
in Your Child's Food

IS ORGANIC BEST? YES. Organic plant foods are raised or grown naturally without the aid of chemical pesticides, herbicides, hormones, and other man-made toxins. The health of organic crops is reliant on the health of the soil in which they're grown.

Organic foods do not include genetically modified foods, which are derived from genetically modified organisms (GMOs), which have had specific changes introduced into their DNA by genetic engineering, such as a resistance to pests. Visit the Web site www.thefutureoffood.com to learn about GMOs.

Animals that yield organic and free-range eggs, dairy, and meats are spared the antibiotics and growth hormones and are fed organic feed and grasses. Always try to buy organic, lean meats and organic low-fat or fat-free dairy products.

If you can only buy so many organic vegetables and fruits, choose organic for produce that contains the highest levels of pesticide and herbicide contaminants.

Most Contaminated (when nonorganically grown) *Choose organic versions of these produce items no matter what.*	Least Contaminated (when non-organically grown) *You can get by without buying organic versions of these produce items if you need to stretch your family's grocery dollars.*
Spinach	Asparagus
Bell peppers	Broccoli
Hot peppers	Cauliflower
Celery	Sweet corn
Potatoes	Onion
Peaches	Sweet peas
Apples	Banana
Nectarines	Kiwi
Strawberries	Avocado
Pears	Mango
Cherries	Papaya
Red raspberries	Pineapple
Imported grapes	

Let me repeat: buy organic versions of the most contaminated vegetables and fruits listed in the chart above whenever you can. If nonorganically grown produce is all that's available, then wash it very thoroughly and peel if it can be peeled.

When buying fish, go for wild-caught, which is much less contaminated with PCBs and dioxins.

How your child's body gets rid of toxins

Liver detoxification occurs in two phases: In phase 1, toxins are filtered out of the bloodstream in the liver; the enzymes of phase 1 detox each specialize in detoxifying specific kinds of chemicals. Once phase 1 has worked on the toxins, phase 2 enzymes further alter them and transform them into a form ready for excretion through urine and feces. To help promote phase 2 detox, get plenty of the following: brassica foods (broccoli, cauliflower, and cabbage), foods rich in sulfur (eggs, garlic, and onion), foods rich in vitamin C (sweet peppers, citrus), fish, foods rich in B_{12} and folic acid (whole grains and vegetables), and green tea.

The liver makes a fatty substance called bile, which soaks up fat-soluble toxins in the liver and is stored in the gallbladder to be excreted into the GI tract. To enhance the detox process, fiber is needed. Soluble fiber like that in apples, grapes, broccoli, oats, carrots, and seeds will bind up fat-soluble toxins in bile and quickly move them out of the body through the next bowel movement. If fiber is inadequate, fat-soluble toxins move more slowly down the GI tract (fiber increases GI motility). Bacteria hanging around in your intestines have more time to transform these toxins into even more toxic versions that can be reabsorbed.

Promoting the flow of bile can aid in toxin removal through bowel movements. Artichokes, beets, dandelion root, and the spice turmeric improve the flow of bile from the liver. By promoting good liver function, chlorella, an algae, is a powerful detox agent; it also helps balance the action of phase 1 and phase 2 enzymes. Spirulina, another form of algae, contains enzymes that can aid in digestion.

Aiding the Body's Detox System

1. Feed your child more broccoli, cauliflower, cabbage, eggs, garlic, onion, sweet peppers, citrus fruits, fish, whole grains, artichokes, beets, dandelion root, and turmeric to optimize the liver's ability to detoxify toxins.

2. Add more fiber to your child's diet with foods like apples, grapes, oats, carrots, and seeds to remove the toxins from the body.

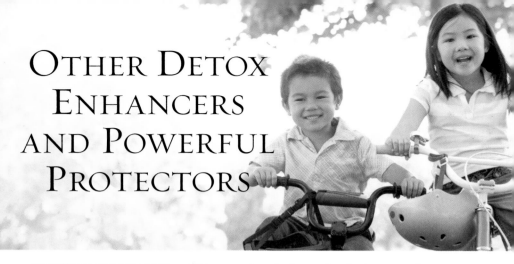

OTHER DETOX ENHANCERS AND POWERFUL PROTECTORS

ONCE YOUR CHILD'S LIVER and GI tract are functioning optimally, there are a few more simple things that you can do to help your child detox chemicals and other toxins.

1. Have your child consume extra fiber, or foods high in fiber, and water to decrease transit time, giving his or her system fewer opportunities to absorb and reabsorb toxins from food.

2. Have your child sit down and relax while eating, which will enable his or her stomach to produce adequate amounts of hydrochloric acid and the pancreas to produce adequate digestive enzymes. Adequate hydrochloric acid is our first line of defense against parasites, and eating in a relaxed, pleasant environment will certainly help. Limit beverages with a meal to only 8 ounces, and have your child chew his or her food thoroughly until it is liquid in the mouth for better absorption.

3. Sea vegetables reduce toxicity: kelp, wakame, kombu, and nori are rich sources of vitamins, minerals, and healing plant chemicals. They contain algin, a soluble fiber that binds metals for removal in short order to prevent reabsorption.

4. Make sure a good eco system of friendly bacteria exists. Friendly bacteria break down some dietary toxins, making them less harmful to the body, and keep yeasts and unfriendly bacteria in check; they also aid in preventing constipation and reabsorption of toxins.

   Numerous studies show probiotics are the single best supplement for prevention of respiratory and gastrointestinal infections. Probiotics may contain lactobacillus and bifidobacterium bacteria and a probiotic yeast, saccharomyces boulardii.

   The dose should include about 10 billion viable bacteria per day for adults and 5 billion for children. Prebiotic supplements fructo oligosaccharides (FOS) from foods such as garlic, leeks, onion, banana, artichoke, and asparagus aid in nourishment for probiotics.

5. Help move toxins out through the skin. Get regular exercise that involves perspiration. Have your child drink water before and during activity.

Herbs to Aid Detoxification

Sulforaphane (from broccoli) is a most potent phase 2 enhancer. Ellagic acid, another phase 2 enhancer, is found in raspberries, pomegranates, and walnuts. The sulfur contained in garlic, a phase 2 enhancer, helps to promote glutathione production. Grape seed extract is an enormously effective antioxidant. Green tea is a phase 2 enhancer and powerful antioxidant. Curcumin is an antioxidant and a potent phase 2 enhancer. Selenium is a mineral that helps detox and promotes glutathione production. Rosemary is an antioxidant phase 2 enhancer.

Moving Toxins Out Through the Nose and Mouth

When mucus is abundant, it could be an indication that other avenues of cleaning—your child's liver, kidneys, and intestinal tract—are overworked. A child who shifts to a macrobiotic diet, which consists of specially cooked grains and vegetables (including sea vegetables), will detoxify quickly.

This causes excess mucus to be formed in the nose, throat, and sinuses, and toxins are driven out of the body. To help your child release toxins through mucus, don't give him or her drugs to suppress its formation. Use natural therapies to thin mucus to help it move out so it can be eliminated:

- Make a nasal sinus wash (salt, baking soda, and water) for your child (or use one already prepared, such as SinuCleanse) or use a Nasaline irrigator to snort and drain.

- Brew ginger, peppermint, or cinnamon tea. They are expectorants, which means they thin mucous secretions and open respiratory passages. Have your child deeply inhale the steam from the tea. You can also try eucalyptus or juniper extract in the steam.

- Avoid or limit dairy products for three months to see if this decreases mucous production. Be sure and supplement your child with 500 mg of calcium twice a day.

AT THE GROCERY STORE

FOOD AND HOUSEHOLD PRODUCTS

FOLLOW A HEALTHY PATH in the grocery store, focusing on the store's perimeters. The outer aisles contain the majority of whole foods—produce, dairy, fresh meat, and fish. When moving to the inner aisles, stick with frozen fruits and vegetables and avoid the aisles that contain prepared foods and snacks. By visiting the outer aisles first, you lessen the chances that you'll load up on snacks and processed foods, and always eat before going to the grocery store. Here are my recommendations on what to buy.

Dr. Colbert Approved

Pantry Staples

Canned tomatoes	Whole-grain pasta
Canned wild salmon	Tahini (sesame seed paste)
Canned sardines (whole fish, bones and all)	Green tea bags (try green tea flavored with orange or lemon if you don't like the taste)
Canned tongol tuna in water	Almonds, cashews, macadamia nuts, pecans, and walnuts
Canned beans (a variety: chickpeas, black beans, pinto beans, white beans)	Whole flaxseeds (for grinding and adding to dressings, hot cereal, etc.)
Chicken broth and/or vegetable broth (low sodium, MSG free)	Natural nut butters (try almond, macadamia nut butter, cashew butter)
Canned soups (MSG free, low sodium, low fat, such as Campbell's Select Harvest organic soups—for those times when you need something quick)	Vinegar (a couple of good types—balsamic, champagne, red or white wine)
Salsa	Sesame seeds
Brown and/or wild rice	Oat or rice bran
Whole-grain crackers (high fiber, such as Wheat Thin Fiber Selects)	Extra-virgin olive oil
Rolled oats, oatmeal, or high-fiber instant oatmeal	Tamari/shoyu (naturally fermented soy sauce)
Ezekiel 4:9 tortillas (can freeze or refrigerate to extend shelf life)	Canola mayonnaise, flaxseed oil mayonnaise, or low-fat mayonnaise
Desiccated (dried unsweetened) coconut	Cold-pressed canola, peanut, and macadamia nut oil
Maple syrup (natural)	Coconut oil
Stevia powder or liquid and xylitol	Stir-fry sauces (preferably from the health food store; refrigerate after opening)
Whey protein powder	Dried sea vegetables (wakame, nori, kelp)
Raw pumpkin seeds	

Breads and Cereals

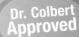

Breads

- Cinnamon raisin sprouted bread—1 slice (2 g fiber)
- Bagel (Sara Lee Heart Healthy)—one bagel or 3.3 ounces (6 g fiber)
- Double Fiber Bread (Oroweat)—one slice (6 g fiber)
- Double Fiber Wheat Bread (Nature's Own)—one slice (7 g fiber)
- Ezekiel 4:9 or other sprouted bread—one slice (3 g fiber)
- Multigrain Manna Bread—one slice (5 g fiber)
- Ezekiel 4:9 Organic Sprouted 100% Whole-Grain Flourless Tortillas (for wraps)—1 tortilla (5 g fiber)
- Multigrain (Earth Grains)—one slice (5 g fiber)
- Multigrain (Sara Lee Heart Healthy Plus with honey)—one slice (5 g fiber)
- Pita, whole-wheat (Sahara)—one slice (5 g fiber)
- Whole-wheat (Earth Grains and Earth Grains honey)—one slice (5 g fiber)

Cereals

- All-Bran cereal—½ cup (10 g fiber)
- All-Bran Complete Wheat Flakes—¾ cup (5 g fiber)
- All-Bran Extra Fiber—½ cup (13 g fiber)
- Ezekiel 4:9 cereal—½ cup (6 g fiber)
- Ezekiel 4:9 Cinnamon Raisin—½ cup (5 g fiber)
- Fiber One Caramel Delight cereal—1 cup (9 g fiber)
- Kashi Vive cereal—1¼ cup (12 g fiber)
- New England Muesli, natural—½ cup (8 g fiber)
- Old-fashioned oatmeal—½ cup (4 g fiber)
- Quaker Oat Bran cereal—½ cup (6 g fiber)
- Quaker Oat High-Fiber Instant Oatmeal (plain or cinnamon)—1 packet (10 g fiber)
- Steel-cut oatmeal (preferred oatmeal)—½ cup (8 g fiber)

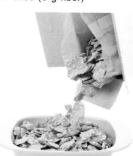

Why cold-pressed oils?

Cold-pressed oils are preferable; other processing methods introduce high temperatures and/or chemicals that can make the oils oxidized and very inflammatory.

FOODS TO KEEP IN YOUR FRIDGE AND FREEZER

Refrigerator staples

- Organic omega-3 eggs
- Lemonade made with stevia
- Fruit-sweetened ketchup
- Organic plain yogurt (low fat or nonfat—no sugar or high-fructose corn syrup; Greek varieties without fruit syrup preferred), such as vanilla or plain
- Apples (organic if possible; if not, peel or wash very thoroughly)
- Organic butter or Smart Balance
- Organic low-fat cheese (mozzarella, feta)
- Salad greens

- Celery
- Onions
- Minced garlic
- Minced ginger
- Lemons
- Limes
- Tofu
- Almond milk or brown rice milk
- Organic skim milk
- Liquid chlorophyll (for adding to drinking water)
- Miso (fermented soybean paste)

Freezer staples

- Pitted cherries
- Mango or peach pieces
- Berries (blueberries, strawberries, blackberries, and any others you like)
- Variety of fresh-frozen vegetables (spinach, broccoli, peas, cauliflower, asparagus)

- Meats—organic or boneless, and skinless chicken breasts, whole chickens, lean pork chops, roasts, lean beef
- Wild-caught salmon, other wild-caught fish
- Whole-grain bread, preferably made from sprouted grains such as Ezekiel 4:9 bread

How Long Does Frozen Food Last?

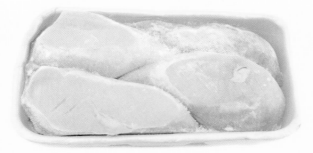

Don't keep frozen fish or other meats in the freezer for more than one month. If you prefer to buy fresh fish and other meats, by all means do so. Having frozen versions on hand as well will help ensure that you always have what you need to make a balanced meal.

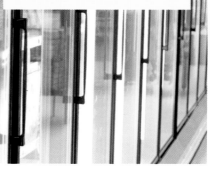

Frozen bread?

I recommend sprouted breads such as Ezekiel 4:9 bread and sprouted cinnamon raisin bread and bagels; just make it something you'll be willing to eat. Keeping it in the freezer ensures that you won't constantly be tossing moldy half-loaves into the trash.

HEALTHY SPICES

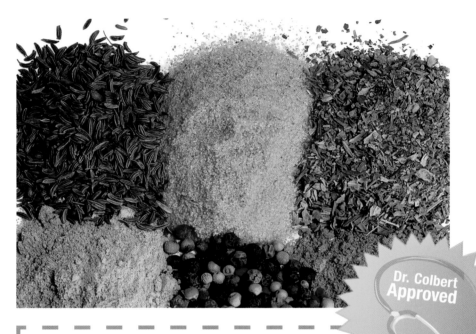

Dr. Colbert Approved

Spice Cabinet Staples

- Basil
- Bay leaves
- Cinnamon
- Cumin (ground)
- Curry powder
- Garlic (dried)
- Ginger (dried)
- Onion (dried)
- Pepper (white, red, lemon, black)

- Parsley
- Rosemary
- Sage
- Thyme
- Sea salt or Himalayan sea salt
- Garlic salt
- Vanilla extract
- Almond extract

Quick Tips

- Don't microwave anything in plastic. This releases toxic chemicals into the food.
- Crush dried herbs in one palm with the fingers or the other hand before adding them to foods. This releases their aroma and flavor. Flavors that are good on just about anything include basil, rosemary, onion, garlic, oregano, thyme, tarragon, and parsley.

Pairing Foods With Herbs and Spices

Here's a quick reference guide for herbs and spices to use with various foods when preparing meals.
Make sure none of the spices contain MSG.

Fish/ Shellfish	Meats	Poultry/ Game	Vegetables	Soups	Eggs	Salad Dressings
Chives	Allspice	Anise	Anise	Anise	Basil	Caraway seed
Curry powder	Anise	Caraway seed	Caraway seed	Caraway seed	Chives	Cardamom
Dill	Caraway seed	Chives	Chili powder	Cardamom	Dill	Chili powder
Fennel seed	Cayenne	Cumin	Coriander	Chives	Parsley	Chives
Marjoram	Chili powder	Curry powder	Cumin	Cloves	Pepper	Curry powder
Mustard	Chives	Marjoram	Curry powder	Coriander	Sage	Dill
Paprika	Cloves	Parsley	Dill	Cumin	Tarragon	Fennel seed
Pepper	Cumin seed	Rosemary	Fennel seed	Dill	Thyme	Marjoram
Tarragon	Curry powder	Sage	Marjoram	Fennel seed		Paprika
	Dill	Tarragon	Mustard seed	Marjoram		Parsley
	Fennel seed		Nutmeg	Mustard seed		Pepper
	Ginger		Parsley	Paprika		Poppy seed
	Nutmeg		Pepper	Parsley		Sesame seed
	Paprika		Poppy seed	Poppy seed		
	Parsley		Sage	Sage		
	Pepper		Sesame seed	Sesame seed		
	Rosemary			Sorrel		
	Sage					
	Sesame seed					

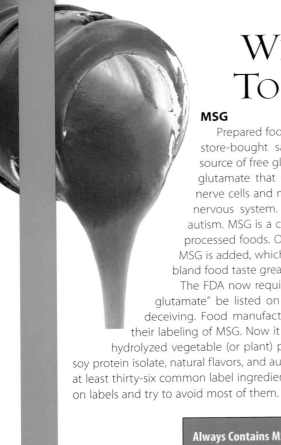

WHAT TO TOSS OUT!

MSG

Prepared foods that contain MSG are usually most store-bought sauces or salad dressings. MSG is a source of free glutamic acid, a form of the amino acid glutamate that acts as an excitotoxin; it overexcites nerve cells and may eventually damage the brain and nervous system. MSG consumption is also linked to autism. MSG is a crucially important ingredient in many processed foods. Once all the taste has been processed, MSG is added, which "excites" taste buds and makes even bland food taste great.

The FDA now requires that the ingredient "monosodium glutamate" be listed on food labels. However, labels can be deceiving. Food manufacturers are getting more creative with their labeling of MSG. Now it comes under the guise of names like hydrolyzed vegetable (or plant) protein, autolyzed yeast, yeast extract, soy protein isolate, natural flavors, and autolyzed plant protein. MSG is found in at least thirty-six common label ingredients. Look for the following ingredients on labels and try to avoid most of them.

Always Contains MSG	Often Contains MSG (or Creates MSG During Processing)
Glutamate	Carrageenan
Monosodium glutamate	Natural pork, chicken, or beef flavoring
Monopotassium glutamate	Bouillons, broths, stocks
Yeast extract	Flavors/flavorings
Hydrolyzed protein	Natural flavors/flavorings
Glutamic acid	Maltodextrin
Calcium caseinate	Citric acid
Sodium caseinate	Barley malt
Yeast food	Malt extract/flavoring
Hydrolyzed corn gluten	Soy sauce (not tamari)
Gelatin	"Seasonings" (when not specified)
Textured protein	
Yeast nutrient	
Autolyzed yeast	

Trans fats

Hydrogenated vegetable oil shortening, chips, cookies, and cake (especially cake icing) or cookie mixes usually contain trans fats. Meal substitutes made with soy are usually high in MSG and trans fats. Trans fats are also present in margarine, many salad dressings, and most commercial peanut butters. They are found in almost every item in the middle of a grocery store--where all the shelf-stable pastries, rolls, breakfast cereals, breakfast bars, crackers, and processed or packaged foods reside. Bad fats are also found in the bakery section in the doughnuts, pastries, cookies, cakes, pies, and other items that entice you as you walk around the grocery store. Try to avoid the middle aisles and bakeries in the grocery store so that you won't be tempted.

Avoid Artificial Sweeteners

I do not recommend aspartame (NutraSweet) because when it is broken down in the digestive tract, 40 percent is aspartic acid, an excitotoxin that may eventually damage the brain and nervous system. (For more information on artificial sweeteners, please see my book *The Seven Pillars of Health*.)

Natural sweeteners

Two safe sweeteners are xylitol and stevia. Here is some more information about both of these natural sweeteners.

Stevia

This is an herbal sweetener with no calories and a glycemic index value of 0. It is my favorite natural sweetener, and I use the liquid form of stevia in my coffee and tea. In this form, it is very sweet—approximately 200 times sweeter than sugar, in fact. Because of this, you only need to use a tiny amount of it. Stevia is also available in granulated form. Products such as Truvia contain granulated stevia in convenient single-serving packets and can be found in most grocery stores. If powdered or liquid stevia is too sweet for you, I suggest you try the granulated form, which is more like the consistency and sweetness of sugar.

Xylitol

Xylitol is a sweet alcohol with a very low glycemic index value. It inhibits the growth of the most common bacteria that cause tooth decay. Chewing gum with xylitol may help to prevent cavities. I have used xylitol as a nose drop to treat patients with sinus infections. It tastes just like sugar with no aftertaste and is a good substitute for sugar for cooking or baking. Because it is a sugar alcohol, however, some individuals may experience bloating, gas, diarrhea, or other gastrointestinal issues when using xylitol in larger quantities. Because it is a natural sweetener and our bodies do produce it, I still recommend using it in very low doses initially to avoid any GI disturbance.

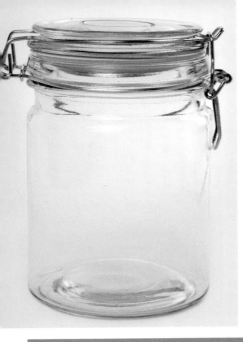

DON'T IGNORE IT, STORE IT!

DINNER SHOULD BE THE most pleasant hour of your day, a time to slow down, relax, and gather with family and friends to enjoy food and fellowship. Here are tips for keeping food healthy all the way to the dinner table. I admit that extra effort is required on your part for healthy storage of food. But I assure you that it is well worth it once you realize both the immediate and long-term benefits for not only you but also your family.

Food Storage Tips

Here are some quick tips for storing foods as safely as possible and avoiding nutrient loss:

- Start purchasing foods that are the highest quality and the most recently harvested. (Organic, locally grown foods are best.)

- If you can, buy your food the day you intend to eat it, or a day or two before. This means buying in smaller quantities so you consume everything quickly.

- If you overestimate and buy more than you can use, freezing produce before it sits around for days is an option, but fresh is still best.

- Refrigerate your produce below 40 degrees to avoid vitamin loss.

- Keep frozen foods below 0 degrees to retain maximum vitamin content.

- Separate fruits that ripen (plums, peppers, etc.) from root crops and leafy greens in your refrigerator. Root crops do best when they are stored somewhere cool and moist; leafy greens (spinach, broccoli, salad greens, etc.) keep their nutrients best when stored in high humidity; fresh veggies and fruits retain the most nutrients when stored at the coldest possible temperature without freezing.

- Don't chop your food ahead of time, as damaging the tissues of the produce speeds up nutrient loss.

- Be aware of which nutrients are most sensitive, such as vitamin C, which is sensitive to air, light, and heat during storage. (See sidebar on the facing page for more information.)

How Long Do Fresh Foods Retain Their Nutrients?

Some people buy fresh fruits and vegetables and store them for days and weeks before using them. They assume that as long as the produce looks or tastes good, it is safe to keep it around. However, the longer the food is stored, the more vitamin and phytonutrient content is lost. (There is one ray of sunshine: Kathleen Brown, professor of postharvest physiology, says that while vitamins and phytonutrients decline, mineral nutrients will not change at all.[3])

Grapes can lose a third of their B vitamins, and tangerines can lose up to half of their vitamin C if left on the counter for a long time. Asparagus stored for one week can lose 90 percent of its vitamin C.

Temperature seems to have the greatest impact on *senescence*, the process in which enzymes break down the food on a cellular level.

Luke LaBorde, associate professor of food science at Penn State University, found that spinach stored at 39 degrees Fahrenheit loses its folate and carotenoid content at a slower rate than spinach stored at 50 and 68 degrees.

Although keeping fresh foods cool is a start, the clock is still ticking. Even at 39 degrees, LaBorde's spinach retained only 53 percent of its folate after eight days.[4]

Stability of Various Nutrients in Storage[5]

Nutrient	Stability
Vitamin A	Sensitive to air, light, and heat
Vitamin C*	Sensitive to air, light, and heat
Vitamin D	Somewhat sensitive to air, light, and heat
Thiamin*	Sensitive to air and heat
Folic acid*	Sensitive to air, light, and heat
Vitamin K	Somewhat sensitive to air and light
Vitamin B_6	Sensitive to light and heat
Riboflavin	Sensitive to light and heat
Biotin, Niacin	Relatively stable
Carotenes	Sensitive to air, light, and heat
*These nutrients are most unstable	

Nutrients Lost in Frozen Foods

Freezing meat can destroy up to 50 percent of thiamin and riboflavin and 70 percent of pantothenic acids, so fresh is always best.

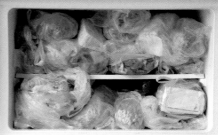

AT THE RESTAURANT

EATING OUT

WE ALL HAVE OUR favorite restaurants, but did you know that some Americans eat almost six meals outside of the home each week? This amounts to more than three hundred meals a year. It's almost impossible to dine out this often without gaining weight and creating a host of other health problems for your kids—unless you commit to sticking with the basic rules of healthy eating.

I've had many parents ask me for advice on ordering healthy food when eating out. When I ask them what they usually eat at restaurants, I discover most of them make wise choices with the dishes they've chosen for their kids; however, they either forget about getting smaller portion sizes or neglect to apply the rules to all the extra things that are usually consumed when dining out. You'll rarely be able to order a perfect meal when dining out, but these are the tips I've learned over the years for choosing the healthiest options possible for your children.

- You can order the right meal and still blow it on the beverage. Save hundreds of unneeded calories by passing on the soda when eating out. And don't think the diet soda is any better. It's not—it's worse! Choose fresh-brewed, unsweetened iced tea, water, or sparkling water instead, adding lemon or lime. Mom, carry a bottle of stevia and sweeten to taste.

- Skip the bread, or just eat one slice of whole-grain bread.

- Request romaine lettuce instead of iceberg lettuce for your child's salad. And ask for olive oil and vinegar as a dressing or a light, low-fat or nonfat dressing (in a mister, if available) rather than high-fat, high-sugar prepared salad dressings. Remember to order a salad with a variety of fruits, vegetables, seeds, and nuts that give you the full rainbow of colorful phytonutrient power.

- Order whole-wheat buns or pasta whenever possible. More and more restaurants are making these healthy substitutions available. Some Asian restaurants are beginning to offer brown rice as an alternative to white rice or fried rice. No more than a tennis-ball sized portion of any pasta or rice should be consumed by a child.

- When your entrées arrive, don't fall into the trap of forcing your child to clean his or her plate. Most restaurant portions are much too large, especially if your child is ordering off of the adult menu. A healthy portion size for most men is about 4 to 6 ounces of lean protein like steak, chicken, or turkey, and for most women a healthy portion is about 3 to 5 ounces.

- Choose a main entrée that you and your child would both like to eat, and split it.

- Try to make at least half of your child's total meal consist of fresh fruits and vegetables. If you are at a buffet and he or she wants to go back for seconds, have them visit the salad bar for more fruits and veggies instead of doubling up on protein and carbs. However, it's best to avoid buffet restaurants.

- If they crave dessert, try skipping the bread and the carbs in the main entrée (potatoes, rice, pasta, corn, etc.). Or try opting for fruit as a dessert or splitting a small dessert order with them.

- Plan what and where you'll eat before heading out, and if possible, eat an early dinner so your can finish the meal early enough to burn off many of the calories before they go to bed.

- Independently owned restaurants are often more flexible with menu substitutions since they are preparing and cooking your food on site and do not have to use prepackaged food items like chain restaurants often do. Keep this in mind as you are choosing where you want to eat.

- Learn healthy food selections from the most common types of restaurants, especially if you know you'll be dining at them every now and then. Most national chains provide all of their nutritional content on a Web site or as a brochure in the restaurant. Web sites such as www .healthydiningfinder.com are an excellent resource for learning about healthy restaurant choices.

- If you are going to be traveling by car, figure out where you'll be along your route when meal times occur. Then, since fast food tends to be less healthy than other restaurant fare, find out where the nearest sit-down restaurants are in that area. Pack a few healthy snacks like fruits, vegetables, and nuts to hold kids over until you reach your preplanned restaurant, rather than giving in to the temptation to find the nearest drive-through when hunger strikes.

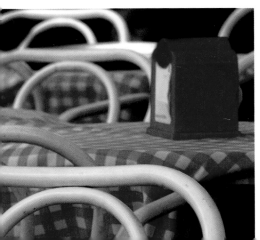

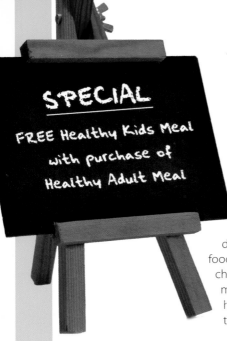

SPECIAL

FREE Healthy Kids Meal
with purchase of
Healthy Adult Meal

Winning the Battle With Fast Food

A RECENT STUDY FOUND that nearly a third of U.S. kids are eating fast food every single day. It's estimated that these frequent trips to fast food joints are adding about six extra pounds per child per year, increasing their risk of obesity. This means that fast-food consumption among kids has increased fivefold since 1970, when most of today's parents were kids.

Finding healthy food choices at fast-food restaurant chains can be a challenge, but that doesn't mean you should give up and let them order whatever they want. If you find yourself with no other option but the drive thru window, here are a few general rules that will keep you headed in the right direction:

- No soft drinks: Order water or low-fat milk for your child instead.

- Skip fries: If a side salad or fresh fruit cup is available, order these instead.

- Hot dogs are not cool: non-fried chicken sandwiches and vegetables are healthier options.

- Be an example: make sure your own food order models healthy choices in both food and drink.

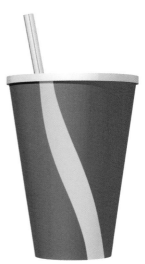

Straight Talk About Supersizing

A 42-ounce Supersize drink at McDonald's is equal to three and a half 12-ounce cans of soda!

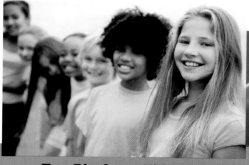

Too Big for a Kids Meal?

At fast food restaurants, the portions you choose for your child after he or she has outgrown the kids meal can make a great deal of difference. For instance, the difference between a small and large french fry order can be 400 calories, a large soda can add 260 more calories than a small soda, and a large shake can add a whopping 1,140 calories. Burger choices range from 280 calories to 760 calories. Are you starting to see how these larger portions can really begin to double or triple the calories your child ingests at just a single meal? A child who eats a 760-calorie burger and a 1,140-calorie shake will exceed their total calorie requirements for the day in the short ten minutes it takes to down these items.

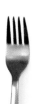

Nutrition Facts

Per 1 meal

Amount	% Daily Value
Calories 0	
Fat 0 g	**0** %
Carbohydrate 0 g	**0** %
Protein 0 g	

Not a significant source of ~~saturated fat, trans~~ fat, cholesterol, ~~...~~, vitamin A, ~~...~~ iron.

Nutrition Guides Have a Big Effect

Parents in a recent study chose foods with 20 percent fewer calories when they looked at the nutritional information before ordering. Ask for the nutritional information on site or go to the chain's Web site ahead of time and do some research on the calorie and fat counts of the menu items before you order.

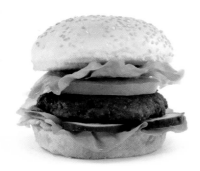

Healthier Food Choices at Fast-Food Restaurants

REMEMBER, FAST-FOOD RESTAURANTS ARE not an ideal option for a healthy eating lifestyle. But in the event that this cannot be avoided, try the following for you and your child at a typical hamburger-oriented fast-food chain:

- Instead of ordering a double cheeseburger (around 700 calories), large french fries (approximately 500 calories), and a large coke (about 300 calories), a healthier choice would be to order a grilled chicken sandwich or a small hamburger.

- Order a whole-grain bun if available.

- If white buns are the only option, throw away the top bun and keep the bottom one. Another option is to cut the sandwich in half and stack both halves of meat between one half of the top and bottom bun.

- Order your burger in a separate container and squeeze it between two napkins to remove excess grease.

- Use mustard, lettuce, tomato, onions, and pickle instead of mayonnaise and ketchup.

- Order a small salad with dressing on the side and a cup of unsweetened iced tea or low-fat milk.

- Instead of french fries, try a cup of fruit.

- Remember, never supersize.

Although most chains have eliminated trans fats from their food, fried foods can pack quite a fattening punch. According to the restaurant's nutrition info, a single extra-crispy chicken breast at KFC contains 440 calories, 27 grams of fat, and 970 mg of sodium. A healthier choice is the drumstick, which has 160 calories, 10 grams of fat, and 370 mg of sodium. Be sure to remove the skin. If you prefer the breast meat, take off the skin, and it becomes a healthy choice at 140 calories, 2 grams of fat, and 520 mg of sodium.

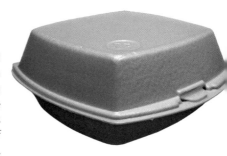

Dr. Colbert Approved

McDonald's

- Four-piece Chicken McNuggets Happy Meal with Apple Dippers, Low-Fat Caramel Dip, 8-ounce jug 1 percent white milk (390 calories, 15 g fat)
- Four-piece Chicken McNuggets Happy Meal with Apple Dippers, Low-Fat Caramel Dip, Apple Juice Box (380 calories, 12 g fat)
- Hamburger Happy Meal with Apple Dippers, Low-Fat Caramel Dip, 8-ounce jug 1 percent white milk (450 calories, 12 g fat)
- Hamburger Happy Meal with Apple Dippers, Low-Fat Caramel Dip, Apple Juice Box (440 calories, 9 g fat)

Burger King

- Whopper Jr., without mayonnaise (290 calories, 12 g fat)
- Hamburger (290 calories, 12 g fat)
- TenderGrill Chicken Sandwich, without mayonnaise (400 calories, 7 g fat)
- Chicken Tenders Kid's Meal, 4 piece (170 calories, 10 g fat)
- Chicken Tenders, 5 piece (210 calories, 12 g fat)
- Chicken Tenders Big Kid's Meal, 6 piece (250 calories, 15 g fat)
- BK Veggie Burger, without mayonnaise (340 calories, 8 g fat)
- Side Garden Salad (15 calories, 0 g fat)
- TenderGrill Chicken Garden Salad (240 calories, 9 g fat)

Choose light, low-fat, or fat-free dressings.

Boston Market

- Quarter White Rotisserie Chicken (320 calories, 12 g fat)
- Roasted Turkey Breast, regular (5 oz.) (180 calories, 3 g fat)
- Roasted Turkey Breast, large (7 oz.) (260 calories, 5 g fat)
- Beef Brisket, regular (4 oz.) (230 calories, 13 g fat)
- Three-piece Dark Skinless (thigh and two drumsticks) (290 calories, 11 g fat)
- Quarter White Rotisserie Chicken, no skin (240 calories, 4 g fat)
- Fresh Steamed Vegetables (60 calories, 2 g fat)
- Garlic Dill Potatoes (140 calories, 3 g fat)
- Green Beans (60 calories, 3.5 g fat)
- Sweet Corn (170 calories, 4 g fat)
- Half Roasted Turkey and Swiss Carver Sandwich (350 calories, 13 g fat)
- Half Roasted Chicken Carver Sandwich (375 calories, 14.5 g fat)
- Half Asian Salad (290 calories, 16 g fat)

KFC

Always remove the skin from the chicken.

- House Side Salad without dressing or with fat-free dressing (15 calories, 0 g fat)
- Original Recipe Chicken Breast without skin or breading (140 calories, 2 g fat)
- Green Beans (50 calories, 1.5 g fat)
- Seasoned Rice (150 calories, 1 g fat)
- Grilled Chicken Breast (210 calories, 8 g fat)
- Grilled Chicken Drumstick (80 calories, 4 g fat)
- Grilled Chicken Thigh (160 calories, 11 g fat)
- KFC Grilled Filet (140 calories, 3 g fat)
- Mashed Potatoes without gravy (100 calories, 3 g fat)
- Corn on the Cob, 3 inches (70 calories, 0.5 g fat)
- Sweet Kernel Corn (110 calories, 0.5 g fat)
- KFC Mean Greens (30 calories, 0 g fat)
- Three Bean Salad (70 calories, 0 g fat)

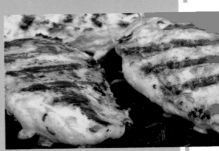

Chick-fil-A

Dr. Colbert **Approved**

I encourage you to eat at Chick-fil-A because they are one of the healthiest fast-food restaurant chains around (all of their sandwiches are less than 500 calories), and also because Chick-fil-A's founder is a Christian.

- Chicken Breakfast Burrito (420 calories, 18 g fat)
- Chargrilled Chicken Club Sandwich (380 calories, 11 g fat)
- Chargrilled Chicken Sandwich (270 calories, 3 g fat)
- Chick-n-Strips (270 calories, 3 g fat)
- Chargrilled Chicken and Fruit Salad (220 calories, 6 g fat)
- Chargrilled Chicken Garden Salad (180 calories, 6 g fat)
- Southwest Chargrilled Salad (240 calories, 9 g fat)
- Chargrilled Chicken Cool Wrap (410 calories, 12 g fat)
- Chicken Caesar Cool Wrap (480 calories, 16 g fat)
- Spicy Chicken Cool Wrap (400 calories, 12 g fat)

Bojangle's

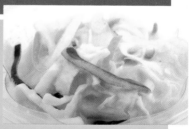

- Cajun Spiced Chicken, breast, with skin peeled off (278 calories, 17 g fat)
- Cajun Spiced Chicken, leg, with skin peeled off (122 calories, 16 g fat)
- Cajun Filet Sandwich, no mayonnaise (337 calories, 11 g fat)
- Grilled Filet Sandwich, no mayonnaise (235 calories, 5 g fat)
- Cajun Pintos (110 calories, 0 g fat)
- Marinated Cole Slaw (136 calories, 3 g fat)
- Green Beans (25 calories, 0 g fat)
- Potatoes without gravy (80 calories, 1 g fat)

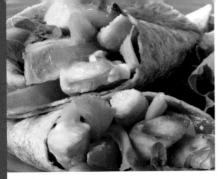

HEALTHY MEXICAN AND TEX-MEX CHAINS

I HAVE FOUND WAYS to enjoy eating at Mexican restaurants by choosing fajitas with chicken. I find that fajitas are a healthier option because the meat is usually stir-fried or grilled. You can also add fresh ingredients like salsa, tomatoes, onions, lettuce, black beans, pinto beans (not refried), and guacamole. Here are few more general guidelines:

- Avoid or limit considerably the chips unless they are baked; still, I caution you not to overeat. A serving is 17–19 chips.

- Black bean soup is a good appetizer selection.

- If salad is available, enjoy a large one with low-fat dressing in a salad mister, if available, before your meal.

- Opt for fresh salsa, pico de gallo, or low-fat dressing on your salad.

- Avoid anything that is topped with melted cheese.

- Beware of sour cream—avoid it altogether unless your restaurant serves a low-fat variety.

- Limit or avoid the rice since it is usually not whole grain. You should not consume more than a tennis-ball-sized portion.

- Some restaurants offer whole-wheat tortillas; choose only two of these if available.

- Choose black beans instead of refried beans.

> **Dr. Colbert Approved**

Chipotle Mexican Grill

Chipotle Mexican Grill uses naturally raised meats free of antibiotics and growth hormones. To save calories and carbs, opt for your burrito or fajita in a bowl instead of wrapped in a flour tortilla. Or ask for a salad and get leafy romaine lettuce instead of rice. You can order many different ways and still have a healthy meal, but only add a little cheese or low-fat sour cream to your order. For more information about Chipotle, see pages 149–150. Here are two healthy options:

- Sample Fajita Bowl: Chicken, rice, lettuce, and salsa (385 calories, 15 g fat)

- Sample Burrito Bowl: Chicken, rice, black beans, corn, and salsa (489 calories, 18 g fat)

Taco Bell

Limit all items containing cheese to only one serving.

- Fresco Soft Taco—Beef (180 calories, 7 g fat)
- Fresco Burrito Supreme—Steak (330 calories, 8 g fat)
- Fresco Ranchero Chicken Soft Taco (170 calories, 4 g fat)
- Fresco Grilled Steak Soft Taco (160 calories, 4.5 g fat)
- Crunchy Taco Supreme (200 calories, 12 g fat)
- Double Decker Taco (330 calories, 13 g fat)
- Soft Taco Supreme—Beef (240 calories, 11 g fat)
- Ranchero Chicken Soft Taco (270 calories, 14 g fat)
- Grilled Steak Soft Taco (250 calories, 14 g fat)
- Gordita Supreme—Beef (300 calories, 13 g fat)
- Gordita Supreme—Chicken (270 calories, 10 g fat)
- Gordita Supreme—Steak (270 calories, 11 g fat)
- Gordita Nacho Cheese—Beef (290 calories, 14 g fat)
- Gordita Nacho Cheese—Chicken (270 calories, 10 g fat)
- Gordita Nacho Cheese—Steak (260 calories, 11 g fat)
- Chicken Soft Taco (200 calories, 8 g fat)

Dr. Colbert Approved

Pollo Tropical

Approved sides include black beans, red beans, yellow rice, kernel corn, garlic mashed potatoes, and balsamic tomatoes.

- Chicken Breast Kids Meal (500 calories, 8 g fat)
- ¼ chicken, white meat, without skin (230 calories, 7 g fat)
- ¼ chicken, dark meat, without skin (180 calories, 9 g fat)
- Boneless chicken breasts, two (230 calories, 4 g fat)
- Regular Chicken TropiChops with White Rice and Black Beans (530 calories, 10 g fat)
- Regular Chicken TropiChops with Yellow Rice and Vegetables (330 calories, 5 g fat)
- Regular Vegetarian TropiChops (580 calories, 12 g fat)
- Small Caribbean Chicken Soup (120 calories, 2 g fat)

Healthy Sub Sandwich Choices

SUB SHOPS ARE PROMOTED as healthier fast food, but you need to use wisdom in making selections in order to keep your kids from eating more calories than they would at a burger place. Here are my tips:

- Make sure you order a 6-inch sub instead of a foot-long sub for your child.
- Order your child's sandwich on whole-wheat or pita bread.
- Hold the mayo and ask for mustard or vinegar and no oil.
- Hold the cheese, and you'll save about 40–50 calories and 3–4 grams of fat.
- Add as many extra veggies as you can.

Subway

- 6-inch Oven Roasted Chicken (320 calories, 4.5 g fat)
- 6-inch Roast Beef (310 calories, 4.5 g fat)
- 6-inch Turkey Breast (280 calories, 3.5 g fat)
- 6-inch Veggie Delite (230 calories, 2.5 g fat)
- Oven Roasted Chicken on Flatbread (330 calories, 7 g fat)
- Roast Beef on Flatbread (320 calories, 7 g fat)
- Turkey Breast on Flatbread (300 calories, 6 g fat)
- Veggie Delite on Flatbread (240 calories, 5 g fat)
- Veggie Delite Kids Meal Sandwich (150 calories, 1.5 g fat)
- Roast Beef Kids Meal Sandwich (200 calories, 3 g fat)
- Turkey Breast Kids Meal Sandwich (190 calories, 2.5 g fat)
- Oven Roasted Chicken Breast Salad (130 calories, 2.5 g fat)

Dr. Colbert Approved

Subway (cont'd)

- Roast Beef Salad (140 calories, 3.5 g fat)
- Subway Club Salad (140 calories, 3.5 g fat)
- Sweet Onion Chicken Teriyaki Salad (200 calories, 3 g fat)
- Turkey Breast Salad (110 calories, 2 g fat)
- Turkey Breast and Ham Salad (120 calories, 3 g fat)
- Veggie Delite Salad (50 calories, 1 g fat)
- Egg (white) and Cheese Muffin Melt (140 calories, 3.5 g fat)
- Black Forest Ham, Egg (white), and Cheese Muffin Melt (160 calories, 1.5 g fat)
- Double Bacon, Egg (white), and Cheese Muffin Melt (190 calories, 7 g fat)
- Steak, Egg (white), and Cheese Muffin Melt (170 calories, 4 g fat)
- Western Egg (white) with Cheese Muffin Melt (160 calories, 4 g fat)
- Egg and Cheese Muffin Melt (170 calories, 6 g fat)
- Black Forest Ham, Egg, and Cheese Muffin Melt (180 calories, 7 g fat)
- Double Bacon, Egg, and Cheese Muffin Melt (220 calories, 10 g fat)
- Steak, Egg, and Cheese Muffin Melt (190 calories, 7 g fat)
- Western Egg and Cheese Muffin Melt (180 calories, 7 g fat)
- 6-inch Egg (white) and Cheese Omelet Sandwich (320 calories, 8 g fat)
- 6-inch Black Forest Ham, Egg (white), and Cheese Omelet Sandwich (350 calories, 9 g fat)
- 6-inch Steak, Egg (white), and Cheese Omelet Sandwich (390 calories, 10 g fat)
- 6-inch Western Egg (white) with Cheese Omelet Sandwich (350 calories, 9 g fat)
- Egg (white) and Cheese Omelet on Flatbread (330 calories, 10 g fat)
- Black Forest Ham, Egg (white), and Cheese Omelet on Flatbread (360 calories, 11 g fat)
- Steak, Egg (white), and Cheese Omelet on Flatbread (400 calories, 13 g fat)
- Western Egg (white) with Cheese Omelet on Flatbread (370 calories, 11 g fat)

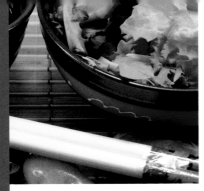

HEALTHY FOOD CHOICES AT ASIAN RESTAURANTS

HERE ARE A FEW general guidelines for healthier options for you and your child when eating at Asian restaurants:

- Instead of fried rice or fried noodles, choose brown rice if available.
- Substitute your serving of rice with vegetables.
- If brown rice or vegetable substitutions are not available, eat no more than the size of a tennis ball of rice.
- Sweet and sour, batter-fried, or twice-cooked food should be avoided since they are generally high in fat and calories.
- Avoid oily sauces such as duck sauce.
- For an appetizer, choose wonton or egg drop soup.
- Avoid egg rolls since they are deep-fried and extremely high in fat.
- Sushi is fine, and some restaurants even prepare it with brown rice.
- Steamed vegetables, vegetable soups, and salads with dressing on the side are also good choices.
- Seafood, chicken, and beef can be cooked teriyaki style.
- Fish can be steamed or poached.
- Be cautious with eating too much rice, and avoid fried foods.

Dr. Colbert Approved

Panda Express

- Mixed Veggies (35 calories, 0 g fat)
- Black Pepper Chicken (250 calories, 14 g fat)
- Broccoli Chicken (180 calories, 9 g fat)
- Mushroom Chicken (220 calories, 13 g fat)
- Pineapple Chicken (240 calories, 12 g fat)
- Potato Chicken (220 calories, 11 g fat)
- String Bean Chicken (190 calories, 10 g fat)
- Pineapple Chicken Breast (220 calories, 8 g fat)
- String Bean Chicken Breast (170 calories, 7 g fat)
- Broccoli Beef (150 calories, 6 g fat)
- Crispy Shrimp (260 calories 13 g fat)
- Tangy Shrimp (190 calories, 7 g fat)

P. F. Chang's

Soups and Sides

Dr. Colbert Approved

- Chang's Chicken Lettuce Wraps (160 calories, 7 g fat)
- Chang's Vegetarian Lettuce Wraps (140 calories, 7 g fat)
- Sichuan Chicken Flatbread (160 calories, 10 g fat)
- Pork Dumplings, steamed (60 calories, 2 g fat)
- Shrimp Dumplings, steamed (45 calories, 0 g fat)
- Vegetable Dumplings, steamed (45 calories, 0 g fat)
- Wonton Soup, 7 ounces (5 calories, 3 g fat)
- Chang's Chicken Noodle Soup, 7 ounces (5 calories, 4 g fat)

Kids

- Kid's Chicken with Honey Sauce (305 calories, 10 g fat)
- Kid's Chicken with Sweet and Sour Sauce (255 calories, 10 g fat)
- Kid's Chicken with no sauce (165 calories, 10 g fat)
- Baby Buddha's Feast, steamed (30 calories, 0 g fat)
- Baby Buddha's Feast, stir-fried (90 calories, 4 g fat)
- Kid's Fried Rice with Chicken (290 calories, 9 g fat)
- Kid's Lo Mein (195 calories, 8 g fat)

Older Kids

- Buddha's Feast, steamed, on Brown Rice (210 calories, 2 g fat)
- Asian Grilled Salmon on Brown Rice (320 calories, 6 g fat)
- Dali Chicken (283 calories, 13 g fat)
- Moo Goo Gai Pan (247 calories, 13 g fat)
- Sesame Chicken (343 calories, 14 g fat)
- Mongolian Beef (337 calories, 15 g fat)
- Pepper Steak (297 calories, 13 g fat)
- Beef A La Sichuan (303 calories, 12 g fat)
- Orange Peel Beef (283 calories, 13 g fat)
- Hong Kong Beef with Snow Peas (310 calories, 14 g fat)

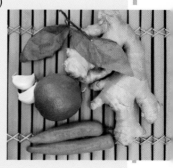

Italian Restaurants and Pizza Chains

ITALIAN RESTAURANTS ARE MY favorites, but like you, I have to guard against unhealthy options. Here are my guidelines for your family:

- Start with a non-cream based soup, such as minestrone or pasta fagioli.

- Have a large salad with low-fat or light salad dressing on the side or use a salad mister, if available.

- Be especially careful with the bread—even if it's served with olive oil for dipping. People think olive oil is healthy, and it is. But remember, olive oil has 120 calories per tablespoon, and those calories can add up quickly if you are mindlessly eating a whole loaf of bread while waiting for your entrée to arrive.

- Grilled chicken, fish, shellfish, veal, or steak is usually a good option.

- Avoid fried dishes or Parmesan dishes.

- Have your vegetables steamed and ask that they be prepared without butter.

- Ask for whole-grain pasta when available, and ask that it be cooked al dente. (Remember, the thicker the pasta is, the lower it ranks on the glycemic index scale.) Don't overdo it; you should only consume the size of a tennis ball. Take the rest home for another meal.

- Avoid creamy sauces, cheese, and pesto sauce since they are loaded with fat.

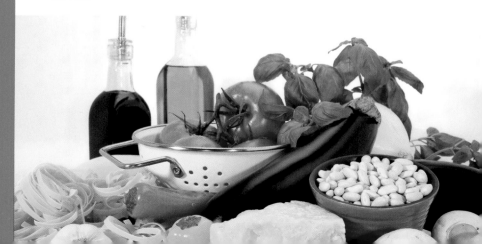

Olive Garden

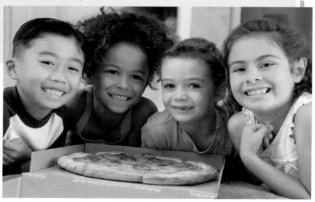
Dr. Colbert Approved

- Children's Grilled Chicken with Pasta and Broccoli (310 calories, 5 g fat)
- Linguine alla Marinara, dinner portion (430 calories, 6 g fat)
- Venetian Apricot Chicken, dinner portion (380 calories, 4 g fat)
- Linguine alla Marinara, lunch portion (310 calories, 4 g fat)
- Capellini Pomodoro, lunch portion (480 calories, 11 g fat)
- Grilled Chicken Spiedini, lunch portion (460 calories, 13 g fat)
- Venetian Apricot Chicken, lunch portion (280 calories, 3 g fat)
- Children's Spaghetti with Tomato Sauce (250 calories, 3 g fat)
- Children's Cheese Ravioli with Tomato Sauce (300 calories, 8 g fat)

Pizza Hut

Before diving in, eat a large salad with dressing on the side. Choose a thin crust with veggies as toppings. Also, request your pizza with half the cheese and part skim mozzarella. Practice moderation when it comes to any pizza. Don't let your child have more than two slices (or three slices for older kids).

- 1 slice medium Thin 'N' Crispy Pizza (190 calories, 8 g fat)

CASUAL DINING RESTAURANTS

THESE RESTAURANTS ARE TYPICALLY high in fats, and the main courses are usually fried. The vegetables are usually loaded with gravy, butter, or oil. Good choices include baked or grilled chicken, turkey, or beef with steamed vegetables. Vegetable soup and a salad (with salad dressing on the side) are also good choices. Avoid the large dinner rolls with butter, as well as any fried side dishes. Choose any beans, including lima beans, pinto beans, or string beans. If you must have gravy, have it served on the side and eat sparingly. Although I was raised on Southern cooking, I have learned to still enjoy the foods without all the gravies and fried coatings.

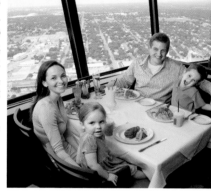

If you enjoy a good barbecue restaurant, keep these general guidelines in mind:

- No skin on your chicken
- Use barbecue sauce sparingly
- Choose corn as a side dish or a tennis-ball-sized serving of baked beans
- Skip the bread
- Order a salad with low-fat or light dressing on the side

Chili's

Dr. Colbert Approved

- GG House Salad with Low-fat Ranch (140 calories, 6 g fat)
- Bowl of Black Bean Soup (290 calories, 8 g fat); cup (150 calories, 4 g fat)
- Bowl of Chicken and Green Chili Soup (190 calories, 5 g fat); cup (100 calories, 3 g fat)
- Cup of Southwestern Vegetable Soup (110 calories, 5 g fat)
- Chicken Fajitas, without tortillas and condiments (360 calories, 12 g fat)
- Pepper Pals Side Black Beans (90 calories, 1 g fat)
- Pepper Pals Side Mandarin Oranges (70 calories, 0 g fat)
- Pepper Pals Side Seasonal Vegetables (35 calories, 0 g fat)

Panera Bread

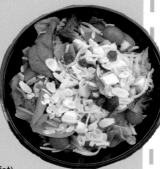

Dr. Colbert
Approved

- Panera Kids Deli Sandwich—Roast Beef (320 calories, 10 g fat)
- Panera Kids Organic Yogurt (blueberry, strawberry) (70 calories, 1 g fat)
- Half Smokehouse Turkey on Three Cheese (360 calories, 14 g fat)
- Half Tomato and Mozzarella on Ciabatta (380 calories, 15 g fat)
- Half Turkey Artichoke on Focaccia (370 calories, 13 g fat)
- Half Asiago Roast Beef on Asiago Cheese (350 calories, 13 g fat)
- Half Napa Almond Chicken Salad on Sesame Semolina (340 calories, 13 g fat)
- Half Mediterranean Veggie on Tomato Basil (300 calories, 7 g fat)
- Half Smoked Ham and Swiss on Stone-Milled Rye (350 calories, 14 g fat)
- Half Smoked Turkey Breast on Country (280 calories, 9 g fat)
- Strawberry Poppyseed Salad with Chicken (280 calories, 8 g fat)
- Half Asian Sesame Chicken Salad (200 calories, 10 g fat)
- Half Caesar Salad (200 calories, 14 g fat)
- Half Classic Café Salad (80 calories, 5 g fat)
- Half Fuji Apple with Chicken Salad (260 calories, 15 g fat)
- Half Greek Salad (190 calories, 17 g fat)
- Half Grilled Chicken Caesar Salad (250 calories, 15 g fat)
- Half Strawberry Poppyseed Salad with Chicken (140 calories, 4 g fat)
- Half Chopped Chicken Cobb Salad (250 calories, 18 g fat)
- Half BBQ Chopped Chicken Salad (250 calories, 11 g fat)

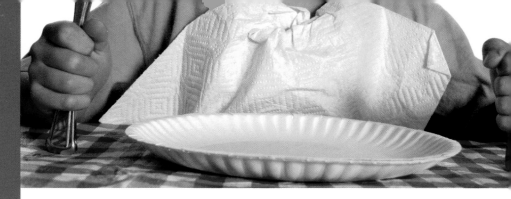

KID-FRIENDLY RESTAURANTS WITH NATURAL, HIGH-QUALITY FOOD

AN EXAMPLE OF A fast-food restaurant that is working hard to make their food both healthier and tastier is Chipotle. Their motto is "Food With Integrity," and the objective is to serve food that is better tasting, comes from better sources, is better for the environment, better for the animals, and better for the farmers. The end result is that they serve food that is better for us to eat. Unfortunately, their portion sizes are large, so be sure to pay attention to calories and fat content when ordering for you and your child. They have five goals:

- **Naturally raised meat**: All of the pork and chicken and more than half of the beef that are served at Chipotle are naturally raised. This means the animals were not given any growth hormones and antibiotics, their feed contains no animal by-products and is vegetarian, and they have more space to move around. Not only does meat raised this way taste better, but it is also healthier.

- **Dairy products with no rBGH**: Recombinant bovine growth hormone (rBGH) is usually injected into cows to increase milk production. It ends up in the dairy we eat and use. Chipotle cheese and sour cream does not contain any rBGH.

- **Using organic produce**: Organic foods are grown without artificial fertilizers, herbicides, or pesticides. This not only protects the soil and water quality but also provides us with foods that have more nutrients, taste better, and are free of potentially harmful chemicals.

- **Produce from local farms**: They purchase produce from local sources, which keeps the food as fresh as possible since it does not travel thousands of miles from the farm to the restaurant.

- **Zero trans fats**: There are no trans fats (hydrogenated oils) in the frying oils. Trans fats increase blood cholesterol, which leads to a higher risk of heart disease (heart attacks, strokes).

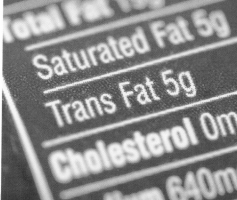

Higher Food Quality
Does Not Mean That All Menu Items Are Healthy

Many of the menu items at Chipotle and similar restaurants are enormous; they are stuffed with too many calories and too much fat. Choose wisely and/or split an order with a friend. The Men's Health Web site "The 20 Worst Foods in America" has suggestions on how to "make over the menu." (See http://www.menshealth.com/20worst/worstmexican.html.)

Other good examples are Au Bon Pain and Panera Bread, which both now use only all-natural chicken in all of their sandwiches, salads, and wraps. There are no preservatives, so you enjoy better taste, lower sodium, and less fat than the chicken they had offered previously. All products at Au Bon Pain and Panera Bread have 0 grams artificial trans fat. Both chains also offer a variety of vegetarian options each day.

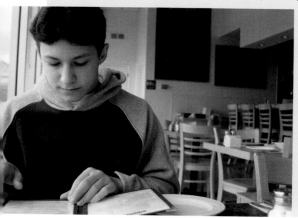

Burgerville and BurgerMeister, regional chains on the West Coast, serve burgers made from naturally raised meat that is from local sources.

SPECIAL DIETS
FOR SPECIAL CONDITIONS

THE FOUR AS:
AUTISM, ADHD,
ALLERGIES, AND ASTHMA

ADHD AND AUTISM HAVE reached epidemic proportions. These conditions overlap with each other. Many of these children also present with ADD, allergies, asthma, eczema, dyspraxia (clumsiness), and dyslexia learning problems. Why are all these conditions related? What underlying problem makes them vulnerable or susceptible to these conditions?

One factor unites all these patients: digestive abnormalities. It appears that the digestive system holds the key to a child's mental development. The underlying disorder, which originates in the gut and manifests itself as any combination of these conditions, is called GAPS (gut and psychology syndrome). The theory behind GAPS is that there is a strong link between gastrointestinal disorders and emotional/behavioral issues. What your child eats plays a much bigger role in managing and reversing these conditions than was previously recognized.

From my own experience, it is rare to meet a GAPS child who is not a finicky eater. The diet appropriate for GAPS patients is largely based on the specific carbohydrate diet, which includes a gluten- and casein-free diet.

So, what's for dinner? Dietary restrictions depend on the severity of the disorder, becoming more extensive the more intense the symptoms. The kind of carbohydrates allowed on the diet are mono-sugars found in fruits and vegetables. All complex carbohydrates should be deemphasized or rigorously excluded from the diet. Anything made from sugar can be excluded. No white rice or biscuits; cakes; pasta; bread made from refined white flour; or chips, popcorn, or ice cream. Since this is all many GAPS children eat, as a parent reading about this diet, you might be concerned that your child will starve.

GAPS children tend to limit their diets to processed carbohydrates because they crave them as a result of their abnormal gut flora. But you can relax: your child need not be deprived of bread, cakes, biscuits, crackers, pancakes, waffles, and muffins if you simply replace wheat flour with ground nuts or nut flour. Instead of sugar you will use unprocessed natural honey and dried fruit. Check the Web site www.scdiet.org for more information.

Did You Know...?

Medical research has shown that GI symptoms like diarrhea and constipation are more prevalent in autistic kids. Up to 85 percent of children with autism suffer from a digestive problem that requires a special diet. An elmination approach may be the best way to get started: simply eliminate different foods from your child's diet for a period of time and evaluate his or her behavior during this time to see if there is any change.

Can Diet Help ADHD?

If your child has been diagnosed with ADHD, a high-protein diet (beans, eggs, meat, nuts, etc.) can help improve concentration. You'll want to help your child avoid simple carbohydrates (candy, corn syrup, honey, sugar) and products made from refined white flour, white rice, and white potatoes. Instead of unhealthy carbs and fats, offer meals with complex carbohydrates, such as vegetables and some fruits (oranges, tangerines, pears, grapefruit, apples, and kiwi), and omega-3 fatty acids (tongol tuna, salmon, other cold-water white fish, walnuts, Brazil nuts, and olive oil).

GFCF Diets Are Key

Diet is the best medicine for treating autism spectrum disorder (ASD). In other words, nutrition plays a major part in the management of children with autism. From my experience, a gluten-free, caseine-free (GFCF) diet or a wheat-free, dairy-free diet appears to be the key. Talk with your doctor about any changes you would like to make to your child's diet so that you can be sure they will not create adverse reactions to any medications he or she may be taking.

Food Additives and ADHD

The American Academy of Pediatrics recommends eliminating preservatives and food colorings from the diets of kids with ADHD. Anyone with ADHD should avoid:

- Artificial colors, especially red and yellow

- Food additives such as aspartame, MSG (monosodium glutamate), and nitrites

THE GAPS DIET

MEATS AND FISH (FRESH OR FROZEN) These foods have the highest concentrations of vitamins, minerals, amino acids, and nourishing fats that we need: vitamins B_1, B_2, B_3, B_5, B_6, B_{12}, biotin. For vitamin A, the richest sources are meat, poultry, and eggs. Vitamin D's richest source is fish oils. Vitamin C and folic acid come from fruits and vegetables. Fruit (except avocado) generally interfere with the digestion of meat and should be eaten between meals. Vegetables combine with meats and fish very well (eat them together); this balances acidity and alkalinity of the body. A majority of GAPS kids are anemic, and the best remedy for anemia is red meat.

All preserved meats and fish must be avoided. They contain preservatives, starches, sugar, and too much salt. Bacon and commercially available sausage and delicatessen meats must be excluded. If you find a local butcher to make sausage, specify only three ingredients—meat, salt, and pepper; that's all!

EGGS Raw egg yolk has been compared to human milk as it absorbs almost 100 percent without needing digestion. Egg yolks provide most essential amino acids, many vitamins (including B_1, B_2, B_6, B_{12}, A, C, D), biotin, essential fatty acids, and lots of zinc and magnesium, which GAPs kids are deficient in. Egg yolks are rich in choline and amino acid building blocks for acethylcholine, a neurotransmitter used for cognitive learning processes in the brain. It is sad that based on faulty "science," eggs have been made unpopular because they contain cholesterol. There is no correlation between eating eggs and increased risk of heart disease.

NONSTARCHY FRESH VEGETABLES These include artichokes, beets, asparagus, broccoli, brussels sprouts, cabbage, cauliflower, carrots, cucumbers, garlic, onions, kale, parsley, green peas, squash, spinach, tomatoes, and others. All vegetables should be peeled, deseeded, and cooked. If any diarrhea occurs, once it has cleared up, raw vegetables can be slowly introduced with meats or as snacks.

FRUIT All fruit can be eaten, including berries. Fruit can be fresh, cooked, raw, dried (no sorbates, sulfites, sugar, or starch added), or frozen. All the recommendations for fruit preparations are similar to vegetable preparations above, except slowly introduce cooked or raw fruit as a snack between meals. Fruit may interfere with the digestion of meats. Avocado is the only fruit that combines well with meat. Fruit should be ripe; unripe fruit has too much starch. All sorts of edible berries are allowed on the diet—strawberry, blueberry, raspberry, currents, blackberries, and elderberries.

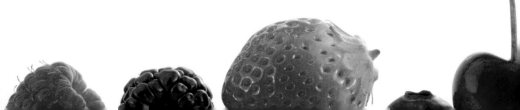

NUTS AND SEEDS These include walnuts, almonds, brazil nuts, pecans, hazelnuts, sunflower seeds, pumpkin seeds, and sesame seeds. Nuts and seeds should be bought in their shells or freshly shelled. They should not be roasted, salted, coated, or processed in any other way. Sunflower, pumpkin, and sesame seeds are best soaked in water for twelve hours or slightly sprouted. They're much easier to digest and are more nourishing.

BEANS AND PULSES Dried white (navy) beans, lima beans (dried and fresh), string beans, lentils, and split peas are all allowed. All other beans are too starchy and should be avoided. With dried beans, lentils, and peas, it's important to soak them in water for twelve hours, drain, and rinse well to remove harmful substances before cooking.

HONEY All natural honey is allowed; raw, unprocessed honey is preferable. Honey is sweeter than table sugar and contains two monosaccharides—fructose and glucose, which GAPS digestive system can handle.

BEVERAGES GAPS kids should drink water and squeezed juices. Herbal teas are allowed as long as they are made from fresh single herbs. Freshly made ginger tea is a good digestive drink.

Water between meals is best; if drunk with meals, it may interfere with digestion.

Freshly squeezed fruit and vegetable juices are highly recommended—they speed up the process and support the liver. Commercially available juices are to be avoided. These juices are pasteurized, which destroys a lot of nutrition and turns it into a source of processed sugar.

FATS AND OILS All natural fats in meats are allowed since they don't change their chemical structure when heated. Most regular cooking vegetable oils contain harmful oxidized fats or trans fats and should be avoided. Natural nonhydrogenated coconut oil can be used for cooking and baking. Virgin cold-pressed olive oil is very acceptable, but only cook with it at low temperatures. Heating destroys nutrients and converts unsaturated fatty acids into oxidized fats and trans fats. Other cold-pressed oils such as flaxseed, avocado, and evening primrose are excellent but should never be heated.

Avoid artificial fats like margarine. Avoid all foods cooked with these fats.

ESSENTIAL SUPPLEMENTS FOR GAPS KIDS These include an effective therapeutic-strength probiotic, essential fatty acids, vitamin A, vitamin D, digestive enzymes, and a whole-food concentrated micronutrient supplement. (See Appendix E.)

ALLERGIES AND YOUR CHILD

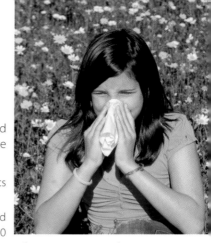

ALLERGIES ARE AMONG THE most powerful and destructive of all the interwoven forces that compose the new childhood epidemics.

- Allergies contribute immeasurably to the epidemics of autism, ADHD, and asthma.

- Allergies are an epidemic in their own right. Food allergies have increased by approximately 400 percent in just the last ten years, and fatal allergies are far more common than ever before.

Many people vastly underestimate the harm that allergies do. They don't perceive allergies as a life-or-death issue, only a minor annoyance that causes sniffling and hives. However, the vast majority of all children with autism, ADHD, and asthma have serious allergies. As a general rule, these three disorders cannot be overcome without alleviating the damage done by allergies.

The incidence of allergies is just as high among ADHD kids as it is among autistic children. In fact, it's extremely rare for me to treat an ADHD kid without finding evidence of a reaction to at least one allergen. In addition, almost all asthmatic kids react to certain foods or airborne allergens.

Sometimes kids who are misdiagnosed with ADHD don't have the classic features of ADHD at all but instead have allergic symptoms that mimic ADHD symptoms. These allergic symptoms can include restlessness, insomnia, poor cognitive function, depression, and hyperactivity. These mental and emotional reactions to allergens are sometimes referred to as cerebral allergies, because their most obvious symptoms are neurological.

Disorders Associated With Allergies

Following are various problems that allergies often trigger, contribute to, or mimic.

ADHD	Eating disorders
Arthritis	Eczema, acne, and hives
Asthma	Fibromyalgia
Candida	Hay fever
Chronic ear infections	Headaches
Chronic fatigue syndrome	Hypoglycemia
Chronic pain	Insomnia
Cognitive and mood disorders	Irritable bowel syndrome
Diabetes	Obesity
Digestive disorders	Sinusitis

Allergies also often mimic other disorders besides ADHD. For example, they can cause symptoms that are extremely similar to those of irritable bowel syndrome, even among people who don't have classic IBS. Because allergies so often mimic symptoms of other disorders, they are sometimes referred to as "the great pretenders."

The most common way to deal with allergies through diet is to avoid eating the foods that trigger allergic reactions. However, rather than eliminating these foods forever, some people find that by reintroducing foods after several months, they are able to tolerate them in their diet, and the allergic reaction usually subsides. NOTE: You should always talk to your doctor before attempting to change your diet related to food allergies. (See Appendix E for more information on delayed food sensitivities.)

Food and Inhalant Reactions

- *IgE Allergies*: These are the reactions that most doctors do recognize. They are reactions to foods or inhalants that involve the immune system's IgE antibodies. They are the only type of classic, "true" allergy, according to the conventional definition of *allergy*. They are relatively uncommon, affecting only a small percentage of all people who have reactions to foods. They are generally the most severe type of reaction, and usually occur almost immediately upon contact with the allergen.

- *IgG Sensitivities*: While technically not classic allergies and often ignored by allergists, these sensitivities are far more common than classic IgE allergies, although they usually have milder symptoms. Generally, symptoms don't become evident for several hours. Occasionally they take as much as a day or two, or even longer, to produce symptoms. They sometimes go away after a reactive food has been avoided for several months or longer.

- *Intolerances*: These are simple, chemical reactions, usually to foods, that do not involve the immune system. Because they don't involve the immune system, they are not considered to be classic allergies. Therefore, they are often completely overlooked by allergists. Even so, intolerances can cause severe symptoms.

Controlling Asthma: The Role of Nutrition

Fatty acid supplementation (i.e., increased omega-3 fatty acid consumption) has been found to significantly relieve asthma symptoms. Vitamin C (a major antioxidant) and magnesium supplementation have demonstrated significant reduction in asthma symptom severity. In addition, the incidence of asthma is reduced in those who consume more dietary antioxidants.

OBESITY AND DIABETES

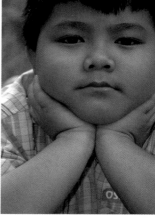

THE WORLD HEALTH ORGANIZATION (WHO) estimates that by 2030, the number of individuals with diabetes worldwide will double. That means we could see the number of people suffering from diabetes worldwide reach as high as 360 million within the next twenty years.[1]

Within the United States, type 2 diabetes is increasing at an alarming rate. Approximately one out of ten Americans age twenty and older has diabetes.[2] And the number of children being diagnosed with type 2 diabetes is growing at an alarming rate as well. Researchers at the Centers for Disease Control and Prevention (CDC) recently made the stunning prediction that without changes in diet and exercise, one in three children born in the United States in 2000 are likely to develop type 2 diabetes at some point in their lives. The prediction was especially serious for Latino children, whose odds of developing diabetes as they grow older were about fifty-fifty.[3]

Why are we seeing such an increase in diabetes? It is simply the result of the obesity epidemic: two-thirds of American adults are overweight or obese, and one-fifth of children in the United States are overweight.[4]

Surely we are missing God's best for us. But how? Many physicians are looking for the next new-and-improved medicine in order to treat diabetes. Instead, we need to get to the *root* of the problem, which is our diet, lifestyle, and waistline.

Fast food, junk food, convenience foods, sodas, sweetened coffee drinks, juices, smoothies, large portion sizes, and skipping meals are all pieces of the problem. The standard American diet is also full of empty carbohydrates, sugars, fats, excessive proteins, excessive calories, and large portion sizes, and it is quite low in nutrient content. This diet literally causes us to lose nutrients such as chromium, which is very important in glucose regulation.

Lack of activity is another piece of the problem. Most children are no longer playing sports and participating in other activities but are instead hooked on video games, computers, text messaging, TV shows, and movies. And they gain more and more weight in the process.

Also, the excessive stress that most adults and many children are under is increasing cortisol levels, and, as a result, many are developing toxic belly fat, which increases the risk of diabetes. Long-term stress also depletes stress hormones as well as neurotransmitters, which usually unleashes a ravenous appetite as well as addictions to sugar and carbohydrates.

Diabetes is a "choice" disease

Galatians 6:7–8 says, "Do not be deceived, God is not mocked; for whatever a man sows, that he will also reap. For he who sows to his flesh will of the flesh reap corruption, but he who sows to the Spirit will of the Spirit reap everlasting life" (NKJV). Most parents and children are unknowingly sowing seeds for a harvest of obesity, type 2 diabetes, and a host of other diseases by their choices of food and lifestyle habits.

I often say that prediabetes and type 2 diabetes are "choice" diseases. In other words, you *catch* a cold or you *catch* the flu, but you *develop* obesity, prediabetes, and type 2 diabetes as a result of wrong choices.

Hosea 4:6 says, "My people are destroyed for lack of knowledge" (NKJV).

High-Fructose Corn Syrup: Sugar in Disguise

If your child has diabetes, you undoubtedly have been told how important it is to limit the amount of sugar in his or her diet. You know you need to choose his or her foods carefully, but food manufacturers can be sneaky. Don't forget to watch out for one of sugar's many aliases: high-fructose corn syrup (HFCS).

HFCS is a blend of glucose and fructose. Glucose, obviously, is the form of sugar in your blood that you monitor as a diabetic. Fructose is the primary carbohydrate in most fruits. Well, if it's from fruit, it's healthy, right? Not exactly. While it is fine to consume small amounts of fructose because your body metabolizes it differently and it does not trigger your body's appetite control center, consuming large amounts sets you up for unhealthy weight gain.

Since HFCS is in many commercial food and drink products, I highly recommend that you stick to the outer aisles at the grocery store and purchase fresh produce, whole grains, and lean meats. Avoid the center aisles, and you will be well on your way to avoiding the risk of consuming a "stealth" sugar that's hidden in a packaged, processed food product. Many researchers believe that America's excessive intake of HFCS is responsible for our diabetes epidemic.

HFCS represents 40 percent of calorie sweeteners added to foods and beverages and is the only sweetener in soft drinks in the United States. Now America consumes about sixty pounds a year of HFCS. The liver metabolizes fructose into fat more readily than it does glucose. Consuming HFCS can lead to a nonalcoholic fatty liver, which usually precedes insulin resistance and type 2 diabetes. If HFCS is one of the first ingredients on the food label, don't eat or drink it. Here is a list of foods that are high in HFCS:

- Soft drinks
- Popsicles
- Pancake syrup
- Frozen yogurt
- Breakfast cereals
- Canned fruits
- Fruit-flavored yogurt
- Ketchup and barbecue sauce
- Pasta sauces in jars and cans
- Fruit drinks that are not 100 percent fruit

FIGHTING DIABETES THROUGH DIET

Prevention of Type 1 Diabetes

In a genetically susceptible individual, four environmental factors may trigger pancreatic beta cell destruction. These factors may render the beta cells unrecognizable by the immune system (they're foreign), and an autoimmune process destroys them. These factors can reduce the functionality of the beta cells:

- Factor 1 is vitamin D deficiency. Beta cells need vitamin D to secrete insulin.

- Factor 2 is cow's milk protein (casein) in the diet. This protein is described as a foreign antigen. An antigen is a substance that stimulates the production of antibodies. Genetically susceptible infants on cow's milk formula have been observed to develop auto antibodies against beta cells of the pancreas; the enhanced immune response to cow's milk protein is the early event in the development of type I diabetes. Children with type 1 diabetes usually have increased intestinal permeability, which increases the delivery of anti-casein antibodies and could cross-react with pancreatic beta cells.

- Factor 3 is that gluten from wheat, barley, or rye in the diet early on may stimulate auto-antibody production against beta cells.

- Factor 4 is nitrates and nitrites. Ground water contaminated with cow manure and artificial fertilizers, along with the consumption of hot dogs and bacon, lead to the development of nitroso compounds that are toxic to beta cells.

To prevent type 1 diabetes: (1) increase your child's intake of vitamin D, (2) reduce intake of cow's milk, (3) limit or avoid gluten, and (4) avoid all nitrates and nitrites.

Prevention of Type 2 Diabetes

Significant increase in physical activity can prevent 30 percent of type 2 diabetes. In addition, a low-glycemic diet is critical for the management of blood sugar levels. See my book *The New Bible Cure for Diabetes* for more information about the glycemic index. Remember, low glycemic is good.

Another good tip to remember: foods that are high in soluble fiber are helpful in lowering the glycemic index of otherwise high-glycemic foods. High-fiber foods include beans, peas, and flaxseed. Acidic foods like lemon or vinegar also lower the glycemic index of high-glycemic foods. A bagel is a high-glycemic food, but if it is consumed with a high-fiber or high-protein food, its glycemic index falls.

Whole-grain pasta cooked al dente lowers glycemic index also because enzymes take more time to convert the starch to glucose; this raises blood glucose levels slowly. So do breads made from 100 percent sprouted grain or sour dough (acidity lowers the glycemic index value). All bran cereal is very good.

The bottom line: if you can't always consume low-glycemic foods, learn to combine high glycemic with low glycemic: French bread with lentil soup.

Nutrient-dense whole foods such as fruit and vegetables are always an excellent choice. The vitamin C, calcium, and magnesium in whole foods are protective. Use a vitamin D supplement, and have your child spend some time in the sun.

Here's a quick list of high- and low-glycemic foods to help manage your child's blood sugar levels.

Low-Glycemic Foods

Asparagus, broccoli, cabbage, cauliflower, celery, cucumber, summer squash, leafy greens (such as spinach, collards, kale, chard, endive), zucchini, green beans, onions, radishes, tomatoes, apples, berries, dried apricots, grapefruit, oranges, peaches, pears, plums, and cherries

High-Glycemic Foods

Tubers and roots, corn, beets, carrots, parsnips, pumpkin, winter squash, potatoes (yams or sweet potatoes are more nutritious than white), watermelon, pineapple, cantaloupe, raisins, mango, papaya, and bananas

DON COLBERT, MD | 162

APPENDIX A

One of the first duties of a physician is to educate the masses not to take medicine.

—Sir William Osler

When I was in medical school, I had an epiphany about the difference between prescribing meds to get rid of symptoms and treating the whole person. I knew that holistic medicine would be the answer to this desire to treat people from a body-mind-spirit approach.

Since I practice holistic integrative pediatrics, I find it appropriate at this point to describe the philosophy of integrative medicine (IM) to you. Integrative medicine:

- Emphasizes relationship-centered care
- Develops an understanding of the patient's culture and beliefs to help facilitate healing
- Focuses on the unique characteristics of the individual person and accepts that health and healing are unique to the individual and may differ for two people with the same disease
- Regards the patient as an active partner who takes personal responsibility for health
- Focuses on prevention and maintenance of health with attention to lifestyle choices, including nutrition, exercise, stress management, and emotional well-being
- Uses natural, less invasive interventions when possible
- Searches for and removes barriers that may be blocking the body's innate healing response
- Focuses on the research and understanding of the process of health and healing and how to facilitate it.
- Maintains that healing is always possible, even when curing is not
- Agrees that the job of the physician is to cure sometimes, heal often, support always (Hippocrates)

Currently, I direct a team of health care professionals who are developing the infrastructure of an actual integrative practice. Our vision has two dimensions: one, a horizontal dimension, which Integrates techniques combining various healing modalities with the approaches of allopathic medicine; and two, a vertical dimension, with reintegration of mind, body, heart, and spirit into the cause of illness and the power to recover from illness.

We encourage the investigation, recognition, and acceptance of the spiritual component in the healing process and the value of both reasoning and intuition in medical care. This new medicine allows us to use new therapeutic tools: nutrition, exercise, mind-body medicine, nutraceuticals, homeopathy, naturopathy, massage therapy, traditional Chinese medicine, chiropractic, aromatherapy, and mind-body medicine, plus other healing modalities.

Alternative therapies and conventional treatments are effective tools, but we need a new map that can teach us how to skillfully use those tools. That map is *functional medicine*, a system of thinking about patterns, connections, and systems that helps us filter a patient's story and emerge with a clear map of how to use all the tools of medicine and healing. In fact, it encompasses all modalities and therapies because it is not a treatment or a test but a way of interpreting the natural laws of biology. It is the map that can guide us through the puzzle of chronic, complex, persisting illnesses that is at the root of our health care crisis. It is heartening that science has uncovered these basic laws of biology that can now be used to guide practitioners and patients. This is the new map that can integrate integrative medicine.

How does this approach to medicine apply to the book you are holding? Because thousands of patient-families like the ones I see in my practice every day need help, they need a complete orientation on this new medical landscape. New information in medical science is constantly updating what we know about disease and healing therapies; however, twenty years usually elapses before the conventional medical community develops an acceptance and general consensus to "approve" the data and apply it clinically for use in medical practice and patient care. For example, thousands of parents and children suffering from allergies, asthma, ADHD, and autism have sought out complementary and alternative medicine (CAM) therapies. A growing number of people have become dissatisfied with drug-based symptom suppression that not only doesn't work but also replaces symptoms with dangerous side effects. Parents with children in the four As will not wait twenty years, and rightfully so. Their families need help now.

If you are reading this book, chances are that *your* family needs help. Above and beyond what Dr. Colbert and I are able to share within the pages of this book, I advise you to seek out health professionals who practice integratively. I suggest you seriously consider any physician who is a member of the American Holistic Medical Association and/or the Institute for Functional Medicine.

I have joined Dr. Colbert in writing *Eat This and Live! for Kids* to be a handbook to help parents in training up the next generation to enjoy living. Management and sometimes even the reversal of health conditions like the four As, obesity, type 2 diabetes, and others can be found through modification of our eating and other lifestyle choices. May this book inspire you to take responsibility for your own health and the health of your child, evaluate your habits, set new goals for healthier eating, celebrate your victories, and take new steps as you journey with your child on the road toward lifelong health.

APPENDIX B

DR. COLBERT ON IMMUNIZATIONS

THERE IS MUCH CONTROVERSY and confusion concerning immunizations in this country. Immunizations have been extremely important in protecting millions of children from debilitating and deadly infectious diseases. Many parents are now concerned that immunizations may cause their children to develop autism or an autism spectrum disorder (ASD). Autism used to be fairly rare with only 1 case in 10,000 children. Now, according to the CDC, 1 in 110 children in the United States has ASD.

There have been theories that the measles-mumps-rubella (MMR) vaccine and/or thimerosal-containing vaccines (vaccines that contain mercury) cause or contribute to ASD, but research has not confirmed this. However, the severity of autism is usually associated with a toxic heavy metal burden and low red blood cell (RBC) glutathione levels (the most important antioxidant in the body). In many cases of autism, there is evidence of mitochondrial dysfunction, which is typical of heavy metal toxicity and low glutathione levels. Also, there is a genetic component and gene tests for autism.

I believe that immunizations are important, but I also believe that we give too many immunizations. For example, instead of giving infants the hepatitis B series of immunizations, I feel that they can be postponed until adolescence. One study has found that many booster vaccine shots were unnecessary since the vaccine immunity was lasting much longer than expected. I have personally witnessed many children who have developed ASD after the MMR immunization; therefore, I now advise parents to have it administered when they are older (at four or five years of age), or as Dr. Cannizzaro recommends on page 168.

Some parents do not want to give their child any immunization ever. I encourage them to at least give their child the tetanus vaccine that is thimerosal free, and many will agree to do this when the child is four or five. I always caution parents to make sure all immunizations, including boosters, are thimerosal free. Many flu vaccines and tetanus boosters still contain thimerosal.

I also recommend that parents give their child a daily vitamin D_3 supplement, 400 to 1,000 IU a day, and to have their 250HD3 level checked periodically (usually once or twice a year). Once the vitamin D level of the child is 50–100 ng/ml, the child is much less likely to develop infectious diseases. In addition, I will usually recommend a quality pharmaceutical-grade fish oil, a good multivitamin, elderberry, and Moducare (a plant sterol) for further protection against infections diseases. (See Appendix E.)

If you do choose to give your child the MMR vaccine, I recommend that you give a glutathione-boosting supplement at least one week prior and one week after the immunization.

Tetanus

Tetanus spores are in the soil everywhere, and you will be at risk of lockjaw from any deep, dirty wound if you live unimmunized on Planet Earth.

Polio

There is not any pool of wild polio virus in the United States.

Whooping Cough

Whooping cough, a pretty scary disease, is still around and may be found in the very young.

HIb

Hemophilus type B bacteria, for which HIb immunization is given, is always around; it is the cause of severe croup, from which healthy kids can die on their way to the emergency room, as well as the cause of a form of meningitis that can produce permanent damage even when treated relatively promptly.

Diphtheria

Diphtheria is another disease against which your child should be protected. In the 1930s, there were about thirty thousand diphtheria cases a year, with about three thousand of these ending in death. The death rate has dropped by 100 percent due to vaccinations.

A Word From Dr. Cannizzaro
Things to Keep in Mind When Deciding to Vaccinate

Immunization is one of the best inventions of modern medicine, and we must understand that it is valuable and should be undertaken on each child. Special circumstances, especially travel, may alter priorities for immunization against infections that are prevalent in less developed parts of the world. I recommend that parents decide on priorities based on the realities of their child's environment and his or her potential for exposure. It will depend on where you live and how much exposure your child has to people, especially other children.

Appendix B (cont'd)
Recommendations for
Immunizations

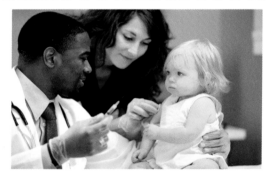

WE SHOULD NOT QUIT giving vaccines, or we will see huge recurrences of these infectious diseases. The first steps are being aware, giving fewer shots at a visit, screening family histories, and listening when parents say that things aren't quite right. I respect the rights of parents to refuse to immunize their children. I do not agree with it, but I will not chastise or criticize you. If you opt out of vaccines, your doctor will probably have an informed consent form explaining what can happen without vaccines. It clearly states that you accept the risk of any adverse outcome of your decision not to immunize. You accept the responsibility and will not hold your doctor responsible or liable.

I do not recommend vaccinating a child if he or she has a fever; has any symptoms of disease, active or convalescent; is on antibiotics; has a past history of any bad reaction or deterioration in health from a previous vaccination; has any past history of an immune system disorder, or has severe allergies, convulsions, or a neurologic disorder.

I recommend parents have full information on the side effects of the various vaccinations. Parents should ask their child's doctor how to identify a vaccine reaction and know the vaccine manufacturer's name and lot number. Parents must report any side effects to the doctor. Always ask for single-dose vaccines, mercury free (no thimerosal). Ask to separate the measles-mumps-rubella vaccine, and ask the doctor to give a single dose (currently unavailable).

The facing page shows a delayed schedule for immunizations that both Dr. Cannizzaro and I feel is healthier for your child than the traditional schedule most doctors and health care professionals follow.

Delayed Vaccine Schedule

Please consult insurance payment policies to verify coverage when alternative schedules are chosen.

Dr. Colbert Approved

Birth	Hep B (only if mom is Hep B +)
4 months	Hlb, IPV
5 months	DaPT
6 months	Hlb, IPV
7 months	DaPT
8 months	Hlb
9 months	DaPT
15 months	Rubeola*
17 months	Hlb, IPV
18 months	DaPT
24 months	Prevnar 1 dose only
27 months	Rubella*
30 months	Mumps*
4 years	Varicella if not immunized already or we can check titers
4–5 years	Hep B series
4–5 yrs	DPT, IPV boosters
4–5 years	MMR if not immune (check titers first)
12 years	DaPT if not immune (check titers first), meningococcal meningitis vaccine

*Rubeola, Rubella, Mumps: If these are not available separately, give the MMR at 24 months.

Immunize with thebooster only for patients found to be not immune. Ask your doctor to check antibody titers to check for immunity. Before giving the booster, accompany the vaccination with cod liver oil three days before and on the day of the shot. Give 100 mg vitamin C twice a day for infants and 300 mg for toddlers three days before and on the day of the shot.

Definition, please...

A titer is a measurement of the concentration of a substance, such as antibodies, in a person's body. Antibody titers can tell your doctor if your child has immunity to certain diseases.

APPENDIX C

2 to 20 years: Boys
Body mass index-for-age percentiles

NAME _____

RECORD # _____

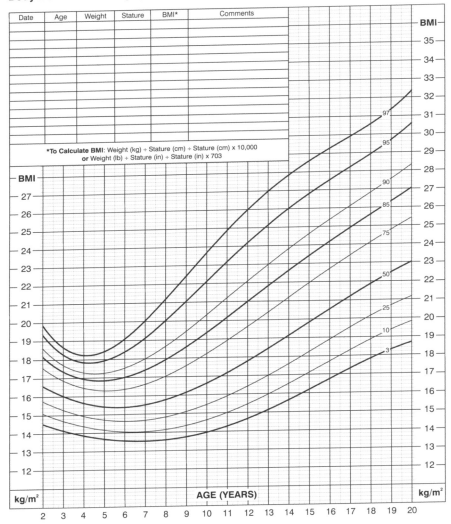

*To Calculate BMI: Weight (kg) ÷ Stature (cm) ÷ Stature (cm) x 10,000
or Weight (lb) ÷ Stature (in) ÷ Stature (in) x 703

Published May 30, 2000 (modified 10/16/00).
SOURCE: Developed by the National Center for Health Statistics in collaboration with
the National Center for Chronic Disease Prevention and Health Promotion (2000).
http://www.cdc.gov/growthcharts

SAFER · HEALTHIER · PEOPLE™

EAT THIS AND LIVE! FOR KIDS

2 to 20 years: Girls
Body mass index-for-age percentiles

NAME _____

RECORD # _____

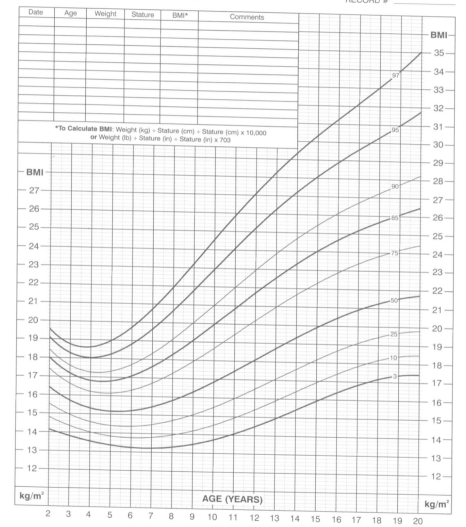

Date	Age	Weight	Stature	BMI*	Comments

*To Calculate BMI: Weight (kg) ÷ Stature (cm) ÷ Stature (cm) x 10,000
or Weight (lb) ÷ Stature (in) ÷ Stature (in) x 703

Published May 30, 2000 (modified 10/16/00).
SOURCE: Developed by the National Center for Health Statistics in collaboration with
the National Center for Chronic Disease Prevention and Health Promotion (2000).
http://www.cdc.gov/growthcharts

SAFER·HEALTHIER·PEOPLE™

Dietary Reference Intakes (DRIs): Recommended Intakes for Vitamins and Elements
Food and Nutrition Board, Institute of Medicine, National Academies[1]

Vitamint	Infants		Children		Males		Females	
	0–6 months	7–12 months	1–3 years	4–8 years	9–13 years	14–18 years	9–13 years	14–18 years
Vitamin A (µg/d)	400	500	300	400	600	900	600	700
Vitamin C (mg/d)	40	50	15	25	45	75	45	65
Vitamin D (µg/d)	5	5	5	5	5	5	5	5
Vitamin E (mg/d)	4	5	6	7	11	15	11	15
Vitamin K (µg/d)	2.0	2.5	30	55	60	75	60	75
Thiamin (mg/d)	0.2	0.3	0.5	0.6	0.9	1.2	0.9	1.0
Riboflavin (mg/d)	0.3	0.4	0.5	0.6	0.9	1.3	0.9	1.0
Niacin (mg/d)	2	4	6	8	12	16	12	14
Vitamin B_6 (mg/d)	0.1	0.3	0.5	0.6	1.0	1.3	1.0	1.2
Folate (µg/d)	65	80	150	200	300	400	300	400
Vitamin B_{12} (µg/d)	0.4	0.5	0.9	1.2	1.8	2.4	1.8	2.4
Pantothenic acid (mg/d)	1.7	1.8	2	3	4	5	4	5
Biotin (µg/d)	5	6	8	12	20	25	20	25

Dietary Reference Intakes (DRIs): Recommended Intakes for Vitamins and Elements[2]
Food and Nutrition Board, Institute of Medicine, National Academies[2]

Element	Infants 0–6 months	Infants 7–12 months	Children 1–3 years	Children 4–8 years	Males 9–13 years	Males 14–18 years	Females 9–13 years	Females 14–18 years
Calcium (mg/d)	210	270	500	800	1,300	1,300	1,300	1,300
Chromium (µg/d)	0.2	5.5	11	15	25	35	21	24
Copper (µg/d)	200	220	340	440	700	890	700	890
Iodine (µg/d)	110	130	90	90	120	150	120	150
Iron (mg/d)	0.27	11	7	10	8	11	8	15
Magnesium (mg/d)	30	75	80	130	240	410	240	360
Manganese (mg/d)	0.003	0.6	1.2	1.5	1.9	2.2	1.6	1.6
Molybdenum (µg/d)	2	3	17	22	34	43	34	43
Phosphorus (mg/d)	100	275	460	500	1,250	1,250	1,250	1,250
Selenium (µg/d)	15	20	20	30	40	55	40	55
Potassium (g/d)	0.4	0.7	3.0	3.8	4.5	4.7	4.5	4.7
Sodium (g/d)	0.12	0.37	1.0	1.2	1.5	1.5	1.5	1.5
Calcium (mg/d)	210	270	500	800	1,300	1,300	1,300	1,300
Chromium (µg/d)	0.2	5.5	11	15	25	35	21	24
Copper (µg/d)	200	220	340	440	700	890	700	890
Iodine (µg/d)	110	130	90	90	120	150	120	150
Iron (mg/d)	0.27	11	7	10	8	11	8	15
Magnesium (mg/d)	30	75	80	130	240	410	240	360
Manganese (mg/d)	0.003	0.6	1.2	1.5	1.9	2.2	1.6	1.6
Molybdenum (µg/d)	2	3	17	22	34	43	34	43
Phosphorus (mg/d)	100	275	460	500	1,250	1,250	1,250	1,250
Selenium (µg/d)	15	20	20	30	40	55	40	55
Potassium (g/d)	0.4	0.7	3.0	3.8	4.5	4.7	4.5	4.7
Sodium (g/d)	0.12	0.37	1.0	1.2	1.5	1.5	1.5	1.5

Appendix E

Recommended Products and Resources

These are products mentioned throughout this book that are offered through Dr. Colbert's Divine Health Wellness Center.

Divine Health Nutritional Products

1908 Boothe Circle
Longwood, FL 32750
Phone: (407) 331-7007
Web site: www.drcolbert.com
E-mail: info@drcolbert.com

Divine Health Living Prenatal Multi Pack

Divine Health Cal-Mag-D$_3$ (calcium for pregnant and lactating moms)

Divine Health Living Multivitamin Powder

Divine Health Living Omega (fish oil) capsules

Divine Health Probiotic capsules, with 20 billion CFU per capsule and Saccharomyces B

Theralac Probiotic capsules, with 30 billion CFU per capsule

Divine Health Infant Probiotic, with 3 billion CFU per capsule

Divine Health Vitamin D$_3$ capsules, with 1,000 IUs per capsule

Divine Health Chewable Vitamin D$_3$, with 2,000 IUs per capsule

Liquid stevia (natural sweetener)

Moducare

Max GXL, glutathione-boosting supplement

Juice Plus

Please contact Dr. Cannizzaro for more Information on Juice Plus, a concentrated whole food micronutrient supplement.

Joseph A. Cannizzaro, M.D.
Pediatricians Care Unit
357 Wekiva Springs Road
Longwood, FL 32779
Phone: (407) 862-1163
Fax: (407) 774-1877

These Children's Natural products are also good for your child:

Visit www.childrensnatural.com to order product.

Children's Natural Daily Chewable Multivitamin

Children's Natural Concentrate Formula (support for ADD and ADHD)

Children's Natural Omega Chewables with DHA (great-tasting chewable fish oil)

Children's Natural Probiotic for Children, with 5 billion CFU per scoop

Children's Natural Vitamin D3, with 1,000 IUs per capsule

The following lab is available to help you with determining if your child has food allergies and/or sensitivities:

Sage Medical Lab, for delayed food allergy testing. Visit their Web site at www.sagemedlab.com.

Notes

Introduction

1. Pam Belluck, "Children's Life Expectancy Being Cut Short by Obesity," *New York Times*, March 17, 2005. http://www.nytimes.com/2005/03/17/health/17obese.html (accessed May 12, 2010).

Chapter 1—Eating Habits of the Next Generation

1. TheHealthierLife.com, "GERD: Obesity Can Increase Your Risk of Acid Reflux Disease," March 29, 2060, http://www.thehealthierlife.co.uk/natural-health-articles/digestive-problems/gerd-obesity-increase-risk-00212.html (accessed May 13, 2010).

2. Centers for Disease Control and Prevention, "Childhood Overweight and Obesity," http://www.cdc.gov/obesity/childhood/index.html (accessed June 29, 2010).

3. Ibid., 3.

4. Frank Mangano, "The Obesity-Hypertension Connection: Your Weight May Be Putting You at Risk," NaturalNews.com, July 27, 2009, http://www.naturalnews.com/026702_blood_blood_pressure_overweight.html (accessed May 13, 2010).

5. Rod Taylor, "The Beanie Factor," *Brandweek*, June 16, 1997.

6. Dan Morse, "School Cafeterias Are Enrolling as Fast-Food Franchisees," *Wall Street Journal*, July 28, 1998.

7. Weight Watchers, *Eat! Move! Play!* 74.

8. Centers for Disease Control and Prevention, "Cancer Among Children," http://www.cdc.gov/cancer/dcpc/data/children.htm (accessed June 29, 2010).

9. Centers for Disease Control and Prevention, "Childhood Overweight and Obesity."

10. Centers for Disease Control and Prevention, "Obesity and Overweight," http://www.cdc.gov/nchs/fastats/overwt.htm (accessed July 9, 2010).

11. Daniel Metzger, "Children and Endocrinology," BC Endocrine Research Foundation, 2001, http://bcendocrineresearch.com/newsletter/v03/n01/Children_and_Endocrinology_s01.php (accessed July 9, 2010).

12. Lara J. Akinbami, "The State of Childhood Asthma, United States, 1980–2005," *Advance Data From Vital and Health Statistics*, number 381, December 12, 2006, http://www.cdc.gov/nchs/data/ad/ad381.pdf.

13. Centers for Disease Control and Prevention, "CDC Study Finds 3 Million U.S. Children Have Food or Digestive Allergies," press release, October 22, 2008, http://www.cdc.gov/media/pressrel/2008/r081022.htm (accessed July 9, 2010).

14. Centers for Disease Control and Prevention, "CDC Study: An Average of 1 in 110 Children Have an ASD," April 12, 2010, http://www.cdc.gov/features/countingautism/ (accessed June 29, 2010).

15. Environmental Working Group, "Executive Summary: Body Burden—the Pollution in Newborns," July 14, 2005, http://www.ewg.org/reports/bodyburden2/execsumm.php (accessed May 27, 2010).

16. Centers for Disease Control and Prevention, "Defining Overweight and Obesity," http://www.cdc.gov/nccdphp/dnpa/obesity/defining.htm (accessed May 11, 2010).

17. Centers for Disease Control and Prevention, "Physical Activity and the Health of Young People," November 2008, http://www.cdc.gov/healthyyouth/physicalactivity/pdf/facts.pdf (accessed June 29, 2010).

18. Weight Watchers, *Eat! Move! Play!* 67.

19. A. J. Stunkard et al., "An Adoption Study of Human Obesity," *New England Journal of Medicine* 314, no. 4 (1986): 193–198.

20. National Institutes of Health, "What Causes Overweight and Obesity?" http://www.nhlbi.nih.gov/health/dci/Diseases/obe/obe_causes.html (accessed September 15, 2009).

21. Pamela Peeke, *Fight Fat After Forty* (New York: Viking, 2000), 58.

Chapter 2—The Basics of Good Nutrition

1. Robert Schneider, "The Framington Heart Study: It's About Your Heart," Examiner.com, March 5, 2009, http://www.examiner.com/x-3795-NY-Healthcare-Examiner~y2009m3d5-The-Framingham-Heart-Study-Its-about-YOUR-heart (accessed May 31, 2010).

Chapter 3—A Healthy Baby During Pregnancy

1. M. S. Martin-Gronert and S. E. Ozanne, "Maternal Nutrition During Pregnancy and Health of the Offspring," *Biochemical Society Transactions* 34, part 5 (2006): http://www.biochemsoctrans.org/bst/034/0779/0340779.pdf (accessed May 26, 2010).

2. MedicineNet.com, "Fetal Alcohol Syndrome," http://www.medicinenet.com/fetal_alcohol_syndrome/article.htm (accessed July 9, 2010).

3. Centers for Disease Control and Prevention, "Highlights: Impact on Unborn Babies, Infants, Children, and Adolescents," Smoking and Tobacco Use, http://www.cdc.gov/tobacco/data_statistics/sgr/2004/highlights/children/index.htm (accessed July 9, 2010).

Chapter 4—Breast-Feeding

1. Naomi Baumslag and Dia L. Michels, *Milk, Money, and Madness* (Westport, CT: Bergin and Garvey, 1995), xxv.

2. WebMD.com, "Breast-Feeding: Nature's Formula for Success," http://www.webmd.com/parenting/features/breast-feeding-success (accessed May 27, 2010).

Chapter 5—The Proper Care and Feeding of Your Baby and Toddler

1. ScienceDaily.com, "BPA, Chemical Used to Make Plastics, Found to Leach From Polycarbonate Drinking Bottles Into Humans," May 22, 2009, http://www.sciencedaily.com/releases/2009/05/090521141208.htm (accessed July 9, 2010).

2. Julia Moskin, "For an All-Organic Formula, Baby, That's Sweet," *New York Times*, May 19, 2008, http://www.nytimes.com/2008/05/19/us/19formula.html (accessed July 9, 2010).

3. Ibid.

Chapter 6—Healthy Habits From Preschool to Preteen

1. Lori Goff, "The Dangers of Stroller Overuse," ParentMap.com, May 7, 2010, http://www.parentmap.com/ages-3-5/ages-stages/ages-3-5/the-dangers-of-stroller-overuse (accessed May 29, 2010).

2. Behavioral Health Central, "President Clinton: Childhood Obesity Epidemic Could Lead to First Generation Not to Outlive Parents," December 22, 2009, http://behavioralhealthcentral.com/index.php/20091222160074/Special-Features/president-clinton-childhood-obesity-epidemic-could-lead-to-first-american-generation-not-to-outlive-parents.html (accessed May 29, 2010).

3. Heather Mason Kiefer, "Empty Seats: Fewer Families Eat Together," Gallup.com, January 20, 2004, http://www.gallup.com/poll/10336/empty-seats-fewer-families-eat-together.aspx (accessed July 9, 2010).

4. National Center on Addiction and Substance Abuse, "The Importance of Family Dinners IV," September 2007, http://www.casacolumbia.org/articlefiles/380-Importance%20of%20Family%20

Dinners%20IV.pdf (accessed May 29, 2010).

5. Jeanie Lerche Davis, "Family Dinners Are Important," WebMD.com, July 17, 2007, http://children.webmd.com/guide/family-dinners-are-important (accessed July 9, 2010).

Chapter 7—What to Drink

1. Environmental Protection Agency, "Where Does My Water Come From?" Drinking Water, http://www.epa.gov/region7/kids/drnk_b.htm (accessed July 9, 2010).

2. Wellness Filter, "The Forgotten Secret of Health: Are You Missing the Most Important Ingredient for Optimum Health?" http://www.wellnessfilter.com/about/TheForgottenSecretofHealth.pdf (accessed September 9, 2008).

3. Barbara Levine, "Hydration 101: The Case for Drinking Enough Water," Health and Nutrition News, http://www.myhealthpointe.com/health_Nutrition_news/index.cfm?Health=10 (accessed July 9, 2010).

4. U.S. Geological Survey, "The Water in You," http://ga.water.usgs.gov/edu/propertyyou.html (accessed June 30, 2010).

5. Levine, "Hydration 101: The Case for Drinking Enough Water."

6. U.S. Geological Survey, "The Water in You."

7. Ion Health, "How Much Water Should You Drink?" http://www.ionhealth.ca/id70.html (accessed July 9, 2010). Also, Health4youonline.com, "Dehydration—the Benefits of Drinking Water," http://www.health4youonline.com/article_dehydration.htm (accessed July 9, 2010).

8. Mayo Clinic, "Post-Exercise Steps for Preventing Pain," Medical Edge Newspaper Column, September 10, 2007, http://www.mayoclinic.org/medical-edge-newspaper-2007/sept-10a.html (accessed June 30, 2010).

9. Beverage Marketing Corporation, "Bottled Water Continues as Number 2 in 2004," International Bottled Water Association, http://www.bottledwater.org/public/Stats_2004.doc (accessed July 9, 2010).

10. Ibid.

11. NSF International, "Bottled Water Fact Kit: Five Facts to Know About Bottled Water," http://www.nsf.org/consumer/newsroom/pdf/fact_water_five.pdf (accessed September 9, 2008).

12. National Resources Defense Council, "Bottled Water: Pure Drink or Pure Hype?" http://www.nrdc.org/water/drinking/bw/exesum.asp (accessed July 9, 2010).

13. Ibid.

14. Ibid.

15. NSF International, "Bottled Water Fact Kit: Five Facts to Know About Bottled Water."

16. John Stossel, "Is Bottled Water Better Than Tap?" ABCNews.com, May 6, 2005, http://abcnews.go.com/2020/Health/story?id=728070&page=1 (accessed July 9, 2010).

17. National Resources Defense Council, "Bottled Water: Pure Drink or Pure Hype?"

18. Weight Watchers, *Eat! Move! Play!* 66.

19. Ibid.

20. American Academy of Pediatrics, "The Use and Misuse of Fruit Juice in Pediatrics," *Pediatrics* 107, no. 5 (May 2001): 1210–1213, http://aappolicy.aappublications.org/cgi/content/full/pediatrics;107/5/1210 (accessed June 30, 2010).

Chapter 8—Supplements

1. The Results Project, "Why You Can't Eat Well," http://www.resultsproject.net/Why_you_cant_eat_well.html (accessed February 1, 2006), referenced in Don Colbert, "Curbing the Toxic Onslaught," *NutriNews*, August 2005.

2. The Silver Gecko Company, Ltd., "About Colloidal Minerals," http://www.silver-gecko.com/extrainfo.asp?LinkNo=21 (accessed February 1, 2006).

3. *Life Extension*, "Vegetables Without Vitamins," March 2001, http://www.lef.org/magazine/mag2001/mar2001_report_vegetables.html (accessed July 12, 2010).

4. National Institutes of health Office of Dietary Supplements, "Dietary Supplement Fact Sheet: Vitamin D," NIH Clinical Center, http://ods.od.nih.gov/factsheets/vitamind.asp (accessed July 12, 2010).

5. Konrad Kail, Bobbi Lawrence, and Burton Goldberg, *Allergy Free: An Alternative Medicine Definitive Guide* (n.p.: Alternativemedicine.com Books, 2000).

6. ScienceDaily.com, "Yogurt-Like Drink DanActive Reduced Rate of Common Infections in Daycare Children," May 21, 2010, http://www.sciencedaily.com/releases/2010/05/100519081329.htm (accessed July 12, 2010).

7. Kail, Lawrence, and Goldberg, *Allergy Free: An Alternative Medicine Definitive Guide*.

Chapter 9—Exercise

1. PreventDisease.com, "More Evidence That Exercise Prevents Cancer," July 2004, http://preventdisease.com/home/tips42.shtml (accessed August 18, 2006).

2. International Agency for Research on Cancer, *IABC Handbooks of Cancer Prevention, Volume 6: Weight Control and Physical Activity* (Lyon, France: IABC Press, 2001).

3. National Cancer Institute, "Cancer Trends Progress Report—2005 Update," http://progressreport.cancer.gov (accessed January 29, 2006).

4. Anne McTiernan et al., "Recreational Physical Activity and the Risk of Breast Cancer in Postmenopausal Women," *Journal of the American Medical Association* 290, no. 10 (September 10, 2003): 1331–1336.

5. Centers for Disease Control and Prevention, "The Burden of Chronic Diseases as Causes of Death, United States," National and State Perspectives, 2004, http://www.cdc.gov/NCCDPHP/burdenbook2004/Section01/tables.htm (accessed December 24, 2009).

6. Christiaan Leeuwenburgh et al., "Oxidized Amino Acids in the Urine of Aging Rats: Potential Markers for Assessing Oxidative Stress in Vivo," *American Journal of Physiology: Regulatory, Integrative and Comparative Physiology* 276, no. 1 (January 1999): R128–R135. Viewed online at http://ajpregu.physiology.org/cgi/content/abstract/276/1/R128 (accessed December 24, 2009).

7. Levine, "Hydration 101: The Case for Drinking Enough Water."

8. Tom Lloyd, study published in the *Journal of Pediatrics*, as referenced in Jeanie Lerche Davis, "Got Exercise? Workouts Better for Bone Health," WebMD, June 11, 2004, http://www.webmd.com/content/Article/88/100005.htm (accessed July 21, 2006).

9. Aetna InteliHealth, "Exercise, Diseases, and Conditions: Digestive," Aetna InteliHealth, http://www.intelihealth.com/IH/ihtIH/WSIHW000/8270/8759/189154.html?d=dmtContent (accessed February 3, 2006).

10. Robert Preidt, "Exercise Eases Digestion Problems in the Obese," American Gastroenterological Association, news release, Oct. 3, 2005, as quoted in HealingWell.com, http://news.healingwell.com/index.php?p=news1&id=528275 (accessed December 28, 2009).

11. S. S. Tworoger et al., "Effects of a Yearlong Moderate-Intensity Exercise and a Stretching Intervention on Sleep Quality in Postmenopausal Women," *Sleep* 26, no. 7 (November 2003): 830–836.

12. Ibid.

13. Associated Press, "Working Out May Help Prevent Colds, Flu: Moderate Exercise Can Boost Body's Defenses, but Too Much Can Be Harmful," MSNBC.com, January 17, 2006, http://www

.msnbc.msn.com/id/10894093/ (accessed July 31, 2006).

14. Free Health Encyclopedia, "Physical Fitness—Benefits of Physical Activity and Exercise on the Body," http://www.faqs.org/health/Healthy-Living-V1/Physical-Fitness.html (accessed October 3, 2006).

15. Mayo Clinic Staff, "Chronic Pain: Exercise Can Bring Relief," MayoClinic.com, August 31, 2005, http://www.riversideonline.com/health_reference/Nervous-System/AR00017.cfm (accessed December 28, 2009).

16. Mayo Clinic Staff, "Aerobic Exercise: What 30 Minutes a Day Can Do for Your Body," MayoClinic.com, March 4, 2005, http://www.mayoclinic.com/health/aerobic-exercise/EP00002 (accessed August 29, 2006).

17. Weight Watchers, *Eat! Move! Play!* 86.

Chapter 10—Creating a Healthy Home

1. Margaret A. McDowell, Charles F. Dillon, John Osterloh, et al., "Hair Mercury Levels in U.S. Children and Women of Childbearing Age: Reference Range Data From NHANES 1999–2000," *Environmental Health Perspective* 112, no. 11 (August 2004): http://www.ncbi.nlm.nih.gov/pmc/articles/PMC1247476/?tool=pubmed (accessed May 31, 2010).

2. Ken Adachi, "Nutrition, the Key to Energy," EducateYourself.org, http://www.educate-yourself.org/nutrition/ (accessed May 31, 2010).

3. Karen Karaszkiewicz, "Storing Food Too Long Cuts Into Nutrients," *Daily Collegian Online*, April 5, 2005, http://www.collegian.psu.edu/archive/2005/04/04-05-05dscihealth-04.asp (accessed September 9, 2008).

4. Ibid.

5. Utah State Extension Service, "Nutri Q & A Chima: Food Storage and Nutrients," http://cindachima.com/Nonfiction/text/Food%20storage%20article%208-05.pdf (accessed July 12, 2010).

Chapter 13—Special Diets for Special Conditions

1. World Health Organization, "What Is Diabetes?" http://www.who.int/mediacentre/factsheets/fs312/en/ (accessed July 28, 2009).

2. Centers for Disease Control and Prevention, "National Diabetes Fact Sheet," http://www.cdc.gov/diabetes/pubs/estimates.htm (accessed July 28, 2009).

3. Ibid.

4. Centers for Disease Control and Prevention, "Overweight Prevalence," http://www.cdc.gov/nchs/fastats/overwt.htm (accessed July 28, 2009).

Appendix C

1. U.S. Department of Agriculture, "Dietary Reference Intakes: Recommend Intakes for Individuals," http://iom.edu/en/Global/News%20Announcements/~/media/Files/Activity%20Files/Nutrition/DRIs/DRISummaryListing2.ashx (accessed June 30, 2010).

2. Ibid.

A PERSONAL NOTE

From Don Colbert

God desires to heal you of disease. His Word is full of promises that confirm His love for you and His desire to give you His abundant life. His desire includes more than physical health for you; He wants to make you whole in your mind and spirit as well through a personal relationship with His Son, Jesus Christ.

If you haven't met my best friend, Jesus, I would like to take this opportunity to introduce Him to you. It is very simple. If you are ready to let Him come into your life and become your best friend, all you need to do is sincerely pray this prayer:

Lord Jesus, I want to know You as my Savior and Lord. I believe You are the Son of God and that You died for my sins. I also believe You were raised from the dead and now sit at the right hand of the Father praying for me. I ask You to forgive me for my sins and change my heart so that I can be Your child and live with You eternally. Thank You for Your peace. Help me to walk with You so that I can begin to know You as my best friend and my Lord. Amen.

If you have prayed this prayer, you have just made the most important decision of your life. I rejoice with you in your decision and your new relationship with Jesus. Please contact my publisher at pray4me@strang.com so that we can send you some materials that will help you become established in your relationship with the Lord. We look forward to hearing from you.

Let's get growing!

Veggies Are Good For You –

a collection of fun videos with great character building themes for kids!

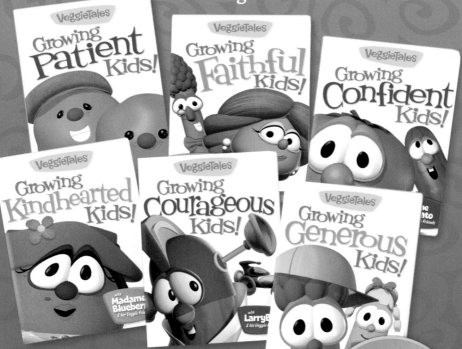

Come along with the Veggies as they teach fun and important lessons that help kids make the right choices as they are growing up!

COLLECT ALL SIX!

BIG IDEA

bigidea.com

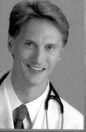
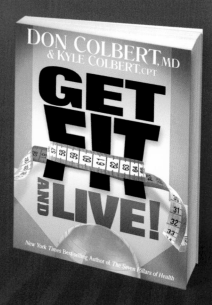
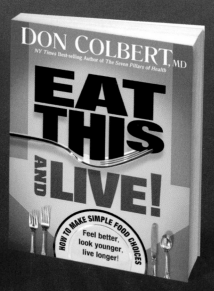

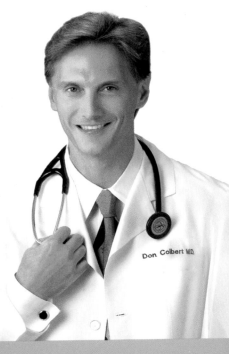
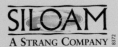

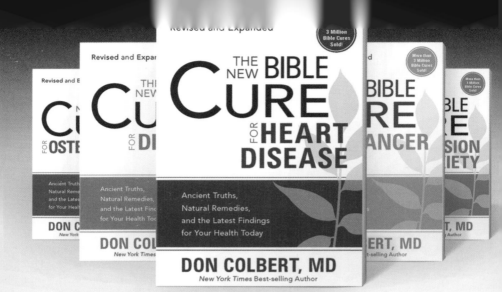

YOU WANT TO BE HEALTHY. GOD WANTS YOU TO BE HEALTHY.

In each book of the Bible Cure series, you will find helpful alternative medical information together with uplifting and faith-building biblical truths.

SILOAM
A STRANG COMPANY
9222B

*PICK UP ANY OF THESE BOOKS IN **THE BIBLE CURE SERIES** AT YOUR LOCAL BOOKSTORE.*